Pharmacological Studies on Combretum Albidum in Thiruvadisoolam Forest

R. P alani

CONTENT

3.11.2	PHOSPHOMOLYBDENUM REDUCTION ASSAY	
3.11.3	Fe^{3+} REDUCING POWER ASSAY	
3.12	PHARMOCOGNOSTIC STUDIES	
3.12.1	COLLECTION OF PLANT SPECIMENS	
3.12.2	PHYTOANATOMICAL STUDIES	
3.12.3	SECTIONING	
3.12.4	PHOTOMICROGRAPHS	
3.12.5	PROXIMATE ANALYSIS	
3.12.5.1	ASH VALUE DETERMINATION	
3.12.5.2	TOTAL ASH	
3.12.5.3	WATER-SOLUBLE ASH	
3.12.5.4	ACID-INSOLUBLE ASH	
3.12.5.5	EXTRACTIVE VALUE DETERMINATION	
3.12.5.6	METHANOL-SOLUBLE EXTRACTIVE VALUE	
3.12.5.7	MOISTURE CONTENT	
3.12.5.8	FLUORESCENCE ANALYSIS	
3.13	ISOLATION AND PURIFICATION OF BIOACTIVE COMPOUNDS	
3.13.1	THIN LAYER CHROMATOGRAPHY	
3.13.2	COLUMN CHROMATOGRAPHY	
3.14	CHARACTERIZATION OF ISOLATED BIOACTIVE COMPOUND	
3.14.1	GAS CHROMATOGRAPHY - MASS SPECTRUM (GC-MS) ANALYSIS	
3.14.2	FOURIER TRANSFORM INFRARED SPECTROSCOPY (FT-IR)	
3.14.3	UV SPECTROSCOPY	
3.14.4	NUCLEAR MAGNETIC RESONANCE (NMR) ANALYSIS	
3.14.5	MASS SPECTROMETRY (MS)	
3.15	DETERMINATION OF ANTIOXIDANT ACTIVITY OF ISOLATED COMPOUND	
3.15.1	DPPH RADICAL SCAVENGING ASSAY	
3.15.2	HYDROXYL RADICAL SCAVENGING ASSAY	

List of Tables

List of Figures

LIST OF SYMBOLS AND ABBREVIATIONS

AO	-	Acridine orange
ATP	-	Adenosine triphosphate
ATPase	-	Adenosine triphosphate synthase
α	-	Alpha
$AlCl_3$	-	Aluminium chloride
NH_3	-	Ammonia
AA	-	Ascorbic acid
ABTS	-	2,2' azio-bis-3-ethyl benzthiazoline-6-sulphonic acid
BC	-	Before Christ
BHT	-	Butylated Hydroxy Toluene
CO_2	-	Carbon di oxide
CCl_4	-	Carbon Tetra Chloride
cm	-	Centimeter
CFU	-	Colony Forming Unit
cDNA	-	Complementary DNA
Conc.	-	Concentration
CA1	-	*Combretum albidum* Frtaction 1
CASPASES	-	Cysteine-aspartic proteases
Cyt-C	-	Cytochrome c
DAPI	-	4,6-diamidino-2-phenylindole dihydrochloride
^0C	-	Degree Celsius
δ	-	Delta

DMSO	-	Dimethyl Sulfoxide
DPPH	-	1,1- DiPhenyl -2, Picryl – Hydrazyl
DNA	-	Deoxyribo Nucleic Acid
DMEM	-	Dulbecco's modified Eagle's medium
ESI	-	Electron spray ionization
ETC	-	Electron transport chain
EtBr	-	Ethidium Bromide
EA	-	Ethyl acetate
EDTA	-	Ethylene Diamine Tetra Acetic acid
FAME	-	Fatty Acid Methyl Esters
$FeCl_3$	-	Ferric chloride
FRAP	-	Ferric Reducing Antioxidant Power
Fe(II)	-	Ferrous $^{2+}$ ion
FBS	-	Fetal Bovine Serum
FTIR	-	Fourier Transform Infrared
GAE	-	Gallic Acid Equivalents
γ	-	Gamma
GC-MS	-	Gas Chromatography and Mass Spectrometry
GAPDH	-	Glyceraldehyde 3-phosphate dehydrogenase
g	-	Gram
HeLa	-	Human cervical cancer cell line
Hz	-	Hertz
h	-	Hour
HIV	-	Human Immunodeficiency Virus
HCl	-	Hydrochloric acid

H_2O_2	-	Hydrogen Peroxide
$HO^{\cdot}$	-	Hydroxyl
-OH	-	Hydroxyl group
IgG	-	Immunoglobulin G
INOs	-	Inducible Nitric Oxide Synthase
IR	-	Infra Red
IC_{50}	-	50% Inhibitory concentration
kg	-	Kilogram
L	-	Liter
MTT	-	Methyl Thiazolyl Tetrazolium
µg	-	Micro gram
µl	-	Micro liter
µ mol	-	Micro mole
mg	-	Milligram
mL	-	Milliliter
mm	-	Millimeter
mM	-	Millimolar
min	-	Minutes
M	-	Molar
mol	-	Mole
Mo(V)	-	Molybdenum $^{5+}$ion
Mo(VI)	-	Molybdenum $^{6+}$ion
MH	-	Mueller Hinton
NCCS	-	National Centre for Cell Sciences
NO	-	Nitric Oxide

N	-	Normality
OD	-	Optical density
pg	-	Pico gram
Ppm	-	Parts per million
PBS	-	Phosphate buffer saline
PARC	-	Plant Anatomy Research Centre
PVDF	-	Polyvinylidine difluoride
+	-	Positive charge
K	-	Potasium
PI	-	Propidium Iodide
QE	-	Quercetin Equivalents
ROS	-	Reactive Oxygen Species
R_f	-	Retention factor
RT PCR	-	Reverse Transcriptase Polymerase Chain Reaction
rpm	-	Revolution per minute
RNA	-	Ribo Nucleic Acid
SSC	-	Saline Sodium Citrate
s	-	Seconds
$_1O^2$	-	Singlet oxygen
Na	-	Sodium
SDS	-	Sodium Dodecyl Sulphate
Na_2CO_3	-	Sodium carbonate
NaOH	-	Sodium hydroxide
$NaNO_2$	-	Sodium nitrite
SNP	-	Sodium Nitro Prusside

SD   -   Standard Deviation

SEM   -   Standard Error of the Mean

H_2SO_4 -   Sulphuric acid

TLC   -   Thin Layer Chromatography

TCA   -   Trichloro acetic acid

TNFα -   Tumor necrosis factor alpha

UV   -   Ultra violet

UNU   -   United Nations University

U   -   Units

V/V   -   Volume/Volume

W/V   -   Weight/Volume

WHO   -   World Health Organization

INTRODUCTION

CHAPTER- I

INTRODUCTION

1.1 TRADITIONAL SYSTEM OF MEDICINE IN INDIA

India is known as the Botanical garden of the world for the reason of well-recorded and traditionally practiced knowledge of herbal medicine. In general, there are 6000 plants were estimated in India, which are used as traditional, folk and herbal medicine. India has indigenous medicinal systems like Siddha, Ayurveda, and Unani that have been in subsistence for some centuries. The traditional medicine system along with homeopathy and folklore medicine prolongs to play a vital role in healthcare system of human beings. Around 7000 manufacturing traditional medicines are found with or without standardization (Choudhury *et al.*, 1998). The modem pharmaceutical industries contain high demand on medical plants. Therefore, medicinal plants increasing the income of country by export, which as industrially important crops (Ganesan, 2008).

At present, people are seeking medicinal herbs as a major source to cure diseases without side effects, whereas the synthetic chemicals are harmful and cause side effects to human health. In recent times, extensive awareness has been generated to exploit the eco-friendly and bio-friendly plant-based products to cure and also for prevention from various diseases and human disorders. In addition, there are 80% of the people around the world have believed in traditional medicine, predominantly plant-based drugs for their most important healthcare (Anonymous, 1998).

Medico-ethnobotany is a new division of science; this is a connection between botany and traditional knowledge of tribal people to consider the aspects of traditional medicine to society. A large part of the therapies consists of a plant extract with their active constituents. India is very rich in medicinal plants and it is continued to be an important therapeutic aid for alleviating ailments of humankind. Tribal people fulfil their needs of plant medicines from nearby forests for curing different ailments. The valuable indigenous knowledge about plants in this area is an important Indian heritage. Tribal are good at the knowledge of herbal wealth and related vegetation in the immediate vicinity. The tribal communities of the area have staunch confidence in ethnomedicine. The use of the plants as medicine has been followed traditionally as trial and error and the effect of

1

plant medicine is being passed from generation to generation. But the uses of the plants for medicine have not been recorded. It is orally familiar to the rustics and tribes. The region is still ethno botanically under exploration.

Hence, it is essential to make the documentation of such important medicinal information. However, many of these potential plants have not yet been studied medico-botanically and its overall medicinal value is ignored. Therefore, it is thought essential to document the medicinal potential of plants of particular region or worldwide. Indian history of medicinal plants is dated back to 3500 B.C. The curative properties of plants have been mentioned in the Susruta of Rigveda and Atharvaveda. Ayurveda has also described a good number of plants with their therapeutic properties. The ancient well-known treatises in Ayurveda are Charak Samhita and Susruta Samhita.

Traditional medicines derived from medicinal plants are used by about 60% of the World's population. Ayurveda is the traditional system of medicine prevalent in India since 2000 B.C. After a thorough study, experimentation and documentation of hundreds of plants over a period of more than thousand years, India's ancient sages have come to accurate conclusions about the efficacy of different plants and herbs. Most of the herbal preparations are free from side effects or reactions. Herbal medicine provides rational means for the treatment of many internal diseases, which are considered to obstinate and incurable in other systems of medicines. In the last few years, there has been an exponential growth in the field of herbal medicine and these drugs are gaining popularity both in developing and developed countries because of their natural origin and fewer side effects (Modak *et al.*, 2007). Many traditional medicines in use are derived from medicinal plants, minerals and organic matter (Grover *et al.*, 2002). Indian traditional health care systems consists *Rasayana* (medicinal plants) in herbal preparations for over 1000 years. Moreover, the medicine practitioners formulate and distribute their own preparations (Scartezzini and Sproni, 2000; Seth and Sharma, 2004).

The use and search for drugs and dietary supplements derived from plants have accelerated in recent years. Pharmacologists, Microbiologists, Pharmacognists, Phytochemist and Natural- Product Chemists are combining the earth for phytochemical and leads that could be developed for the treatment of various diseases. In fact, many modern drugs have been derived from a plant. A lack of standardization of herbal remedies also makes it challenging to understand that causes adverse interactions. Contamination or mix-identification of an herbal plant or any incorrectly substituted plant all raise the issue of quality and can result potentially in an unwanted side effect. The ethnopharmacological use of herbal remedies for the treatment of diabetes mellitus is an area of study ripens with potential as a starting point in the development of alternative, inexpensive therapies for treating the disease. There are over 30 million people today suffering from one form of diabetes or another and the numbers are increasing in rural and poor populations throughout the world.

India is the largest producer of medicinal herbs and is called a botanical garden of the world (Seth and Sharma, 2004). India has 12 mega biodiversity regions which consists of 47,513 plant species, among this 17,527 are angiosperms includes 4,000 medicinal plant species (Cox and Moore, 1993; Karthikeyan, 2009; Singh and Dash, 2014). India has been one of the pioneers in the development and practice of well-documented indigenous systems of medicine, particularly Ayurveda, Siddha, and Unani. For millennia, the Indian population has depended mainly upon plant-based crude drugs for a variety of ailments. This alternative system of medicine is gaining increasing popularity worldwide.

The medicinal plants sector occupied an important position in traditional, socio-cultural, spiritual and medicinal arena of rural and tribal people. Indian government, due to the importance of medicinal plants, started Department of Indian System of Medicine and Homoeopathy. Today, the medicinal plants engage a constant position in new medicine system and also the pharmaceutical industries showing great attention in using natural substances extracted from the plants. Therefore, the demands for more and more drugs from plant sources are increasing from the developing countries. All over the world, people has vast requirement on traditional medicine, because of various advantages such as direct therapeutic agent, lesser side effects, raw material base for more multifaceted semi-synthetic chemical compounds, easily affordable by the people, reproduction of new synthetic compounds, taxonomic markers for finding of new compounds, phytol-medicines, renewable source, production, consumption and international trade of medicinal plants (Samy and Gopalakrishnakone, 2007).

Plants have variety of bioactive metabolic compounds such as flavonoids, alkaloids, phenols, steroids, dyes, terpenes, hormones, pharmaceuticals, pigments, drugs and many other compounds. A wide diverse of secondary metabolites from plants have some ecological role like pollinator attractant, chemical defence against insects, predators and microorganism, and also protect from biotic stresses such as temperature, water stress, nutrition and UV. Hence, the plants are widely exploited leading to a decrease in their availability (Bhojwani and Razdan, 1996).

Since the medicinal plants are the most important source of life-saving drugs for the majority of the world's population, the biotechnological tools are important to select, multiply and conserve the critical genotypes of medicinal plants. *In vitro* regeneration and genetic transformations holds tremendous potential for the production of high-quality plant-based medicine. With micro propagation, the multiplication rate is greatly increased, which is also permits the production of pathogen-free material. Micropropagation of various plant species, including several medicinal plants have been reported. Propagation from existing meristems, yields plants that are genetically identical to the donor plants. Plant regeneration from the shoot and stem meristems has yielded encouraging results in medicinal plants like *Catharanthus roseus, Cinchona ledgeriana, Digitalis* spp., *Rehmannia glutinosa, Rauvolfia serpentine* and *Isoplexis canariensis* (Perez-Bermudez *et al.*, 2002).

For many years, man has been dependent on plants for their life activities. Habitat destruction, overexploitation, and climate change have markedly increased the rate of demonise of medicinal plants from their local niches. It is anticipated that the global warming and climate change may alter the production of secondary metabolites, which constitute active medicinal principles in these plants. Regrettably, only a few medicinal plants are being cultivated on a commercial scale with a majority still being collected from the wild. Therefore, an urgent requirement for large-scale cultivation of authentic plant material whose yield and potency of active principles are known. Large-scale cultivation of medicinal plants would require a thorough understanding of their cytological, embryological, phytochemical and agronomical aspects. Further, conservation and commercial cultivation of medicinal plants would require quality planting material on a large scale, so *in vitro* responses of the plant require to be worked out. Secondary metabolite production in cell suspension cultures and bioreactors where feasible, require to be developed as a conservation strategy.

Since, India is the richest biodiversity region in the world, the flora and fauna is remarkably very huge in numbers when compared to neighbouring countries. Though many plants information is documented, various research agencies and institutional researchers are working to report to cover all the plants in various parts of the county. Most of the reported plants are used for various ailments, based on the practices the plants are used time immemorial in the human settlements. Due to the modernization, human and livestock are affected for various illnesses and it creates a huge demand for drugs. The synthetic compounds are also addressing the demands simultaneously, which creates new side effects too. Thus, the researchers and pharma industries are trying to find new compounds from plants to better use and avoid the side effects. Modern researchers are looking back to the ancient scripts and collecting information's from the traditional herbal healers, this kind of approach is named as "Reverse biology", based on this concept the person can easily get data and also the active molecule information.

1.2 ETHNOBOTANY AND HERBAL HEALERS

Ethnobotany is the part of biological science, which deals with plants, diseases, and humans. The term Ethnobotany was coined by John William Harshberger (Harshberger, 1896). This evolved into a separate discipline in recent decades. It looks people - plant relationships in a multidisciplinary approach like ecology, economic botany, pharmacology, public health and other allied sciences (Balick and Cox 1996). The World Health Organization (WHO) reported that 80% of the world's populations depend on traditional medicine for their initial curative requirements (Azaizeh *et al.*, 2003). The development of native medicines gives significant economic benefits to human beings.

A large amount of information on medicinal plants is collected by Ethnobotanical surveys. Collecting information and documentation is more useful for the conservations and proper utilization of the plant resources (Muthu *et al.*, 2006). These kinds of documents are more valuable for the modern investigators, which provide a brief backdrop to find the disease curing potential molecule from any plant (Smita *et al.*, 2013). Martin (1995) pointed out four major interconnected things in ethnobotany such as knowledge about medicinal plants and their documentation, utilization and management of flora and fauna, bioactive components of plants for subsistence and commercial aspects, ecological knowledge and resources of local people.

In the modern world, synthetic drug usage is remarkably very high, though medical science reached the next level, still the people are practicing the traditional plant-based ailments. These groups of people are collectively named Herbal Healers, herbal doctors, nattu vaithiyar, maruthuvachi (if female), 90% of the herbalist is male; very few women are practicing. Old age healers are not ready to disclose their usage secrets. Due to development of allopathic medicine, the traditional healing methods are slowly disappearing from the population. However, a very small group of people or settlements are still practicing the same, those groups of peoples are categorized as Tribal's according to the demographic census of India.

In India, Tribal people have enormous knowledge about medicinal plants and their ailment values. Almost 68 million tribal people belonging to 573 tribal communities, 227 ethnic groups in different part of the country (Pushpagandhan, 1994). Tribal people will give substantial information about many plants or plant parts used as a remedy for numerous illnesses. The tribal people identify the medicinally important plants by word of mouth or comparison or by experimentation. The real custodians of nature's wealth and experts are tribal people. Ethnic people used undomesticated plants for their curative needs and also they have a number of secrets for ethno medicine. These secrets passed through younger generations. These kinds of databases serve a vital role in finding new active compounds in the modern curative system.

1.3 CHEMICAL CONSTITUENTS OF MEDICINAL PLANTS

Phytochemical is a word derived from Greek, which denotes as Phyto is known as a plant. All the plants contain metabolites, commonly known as phytochemicals, which can be classified by their biosynthetic origin, chemical class and functional groups into primary and secondary metabolites (Pandith, 2012). These components have an effective role in plant life to maintenance and development of physiological functions and induce defence mechanisms against various biotic factors including virus, bacteria, fungi, insects and also from herbivores (Schultz, 2002). The plant produces secondary metabolites such as alkaloids, saponins, flavonoids, glycosides, essential oils, quinines, phenols, terpenes, tannins, steroids, etc. These secondary metabolites are contains tremendous biological activities that promote very essential and play a important role as it human health effects (Saxena, 2001).

Plant scientists have great attention on phytochemicals to develop new and sophisticated techniques to analyse and identify the compounds. This kind of technology plays a vital role in solving the systematic problems in one part and another part finding the supplementary resources of raw materials for the pharmaceutical industry (Mojab *et al.*, 2003). In the current scenario, there are 120 active compounds isolated from higher plants that are used in modern medicine. The derived compounds from plants contain an 80 percent positive correlation between their modern therapeutic and traditional medicinal use (Fabricant, 2001). The researchers from the pharmaceutical field know the concept of drug synergism and the clinical trials are used to identify the effectiveness of concerned herbal preparation and provided the formulation of the herb in consistent manner (Izhaki and Emodin, 2002).

Several phytochemicals were isolated and identified by various researchers time to time, these phytochemicals have important role on various pharmacological properties such as antidiabetic, anti-inflammatory, antirheumatic, anticancerous, antioxidant, antiproliferative, antimicrobial, hypocholesterolemic, antithrombotic, antihepatotoxic, antityrosinase, antiviral, antidiarrheal, carminative, hypotensive, diuretic, insecticidal, larvicidal, antivenomous and cyclooxygenase-1 inhibitory activities (Wilson *et al.*, 2005; Reanmongkol *et al.*, 2006; Chen *et al.*, 2008b; Afzal *et al.*, 2013; Krup *et al.*, 2013; Angel *et al.*, 2014; Sikha *et al.*, 2015; Herath *et al.*, 2017).

1.4 ANTIBACTERIAL AGENTS

Bacteria are the important microorganisms in the biosphere, which can't be seen by the naked eye. Bacteria cause diseases in plants, animals and humans are known as pathogenic bacteria. In anticipation of the discovery of antibiotics like penicillin and sulfa drugs as well as the toxic arsenic, the only means of fighting infectious diseases were plant extracts of different sorts, though their usage yielded various results (Dar *et al.*, 2016; Górniak *et al.*, 2018). Moreover, in the last few decades antibiotics are most important to treat infectious diseases caused by bacteria. Even though, the presence of antibiotic-resistant and threatened bacteria has been observed to increase in frequency, due to their resistance to new antibiotic drugs.

Plant and microbial products inhabit the most of antimicrobial compounds discovered until now (Berdy, 2005). Plants produce complex and structurally diverse compounds such as essential oils, peptides, amino acids, phenols, flavonoids, terpenoids, etc., are as potential antimicrobial agents (Runyoro *et al.*, 2006; Mabona *et al.*, 2013; Nazzaro *et al.*, 2013). The anti-microbial effect of the plant products is difficult to compare their results due to different non-standardized approaches, inoculum preparation techniques, inoculum size, culture medium, incubation time and temperature (Balouiri *et al.*, 2016). The drug resistance bacteria can be accomplished by various mechanisms, therefore to control the problem is a very difficult task for researchers (Saleem *et al.*, 2010). Therefore, the progress in the development of antibacterial agents is required to isolate a new antibacterial agent due to the development of multidrug-resistant bacteria. Therefore, the plants are believed to be giving effective antimicrobial compounds with minimum or without side effects to human.

1.5 THE ROLE OF ANTIOXIDANTS FROM PLANTS

Oxidation is the process of transferring the electrons from one atom to another atom, which corresponds to an essential part of aerobic life and human metabolism. In view of the fact, the oxygen is the crucial electron acceptor in the electron flow system that generates energy in the structure of ATP (Davies, 1995; Gulcin, 2011). On the other hand, the free radicals are generated from the process that occurs at the time of electron flow and develops into the transfer of unpaired single electrons. The oxygen-centered free radicals are known as ROS (reactive oxygen species) which incorporate with hydroxyl (HO), superoxide (O_2 -), nitric oxide (NO), alkoxyl (RO) and peroxyl (ROO) (Ames *et al.*, 1993). In addition to these ROS radicals in living organisms, there are other ROS known radicals such as the singlet oxygen ($_1O$), hydrogen peroxide (H_2O_2), and hypochlorous acid (HOCl) also reported to be generated (Pietta, 2000).

ROS spontaneously produced by standard use of oxygen like respiration and a number of cell-mediated immune functions (Gulcin, 2006). ROS can rapidly generated during the normal physiological events and also starts the peroxidation of membrane lipids without trouble, which leads to the accumulation of lipid peroxides (Gulcin, 2010). ROS at physiological mediation is required to normal cell function, otherwise the essential biomolecules like proteins, lipids, carbohydrates, nucleic acids, and polyunsaturated fatty acids and in addition, it may cause DNA damage that can lead to mutations. In such a way, the ROS are not effectively scavenged by cellular constituents, which encourages the free-radical chain reactions consequently and damaging the cellular bio molecules including such as nucleic acids, proteins and lipids which leads to metabolic disorders or diseases (Halliwell and Gutteridge, 1990).

The destructive property of oxidants and free radicals in the human body was defended by a complex system of natural enzymatic and non-enzymatic antioxidants (Alam *et al.*, 2013). The higher concentration of free radicals in cells or tissues may result in oxidative stress. It was induced by a high concentration of free radicals in cells and tissues, which also can be induced by different negative factors like X-ray, UV and gamma radiation, psychological stress, contaminated food, smoking, drug addiction, adverse environmental conditions, alcoholism, and intensive physical exertion (Yashin *et al.*, 2017). The chronic stress or free radicals are most important factor to origin of various number of diseases including Parkinson's disease, cardiovascular disease, Alzheimer's disease, neural disorders, mild cognitive impairment, cancer, alcohol-induced liver disease, ulcerative colitis, atherosclerosis and aging (Shah and Channon, 2004; Uttara *et al.*, 2009; Niki, 2011; Kumar *et al.*, 2012; Ríos-Arrabal *et al.*, 2013; Gladyshev, 2014; Peña-Bautista *et al.*, 2019). Antioxidants are such type of chemical compounds that can interrupt the initiation of a lipid oxidation reaction in food systems and other biological reaction that leads to metabolic disorders.

The synthetic antioxidants such as butylated hydroxytoluene (BHT), butylated hydroxyanisole (BHA), propyl gallate (PG) and tert-butylhydroquinone (TBHQ) are commonly used in the food and pharmacological industries. Synthetic antioxidants are restricted by legislative rules because of highly toxic and carcinogenic effects (Sherwin, 1990). Hence, researchers are interested to isolate natural and safer antioxidants for food applications. Moreover, consumers are giving more preferences towards natural antioxidants; these things can provide greater energy towards the challenge and explore natural sources of antioxidants (Gulcin, 2007). Nowadays, aromatic plants are extensively used as a nutritional supplement and also a good source of natural antioxidants (Tiwari *et al.*, 2009; Stankovic, *et al.*, 2016). The natural antioxidants, especially plants have a major contribution to alternate synthetic antioxidants due to exploitation of low cost and safer against side effects. The polyphenol compounds from plants are a most important source of antioxidant due to their redox properties, which can absorbing and neutralizing free radicals, quenching singlet and triplet oxygen and decomposing peroxides (Zheng and Wang, 2001). Hence, the present study was intended to isolate a natural antioxidant from medicinal plants and study it effects.

1.6 ANTI-INFLAMMATORY STUDY

Inflammation is a most significant physiological response, which is caused by various injurious agents such as physical trauma, bacterial infection, chemicals or any other phenomenon. The inflammation finally acts dual function of limiting damage and inducing tissue repair (Nathan, 2002). Inflammatory processes are necessary for immune surveillance, regeneration after injury and optimal repair of cells and tissues (Vodovotz *et al.*, 2008). This process saves our system from various diseases through discharging cells and mediators that struggle against foreign materials and prevent infections (El-Gamal *et al.*, 2010).

Inflammation is the most important component that the damage was caused by autoimmune diseases and also primary donor of various infectious and non-infectious diseases like cancer, rheumatoid arthritis, cardiovascular disease, Alzheimer's, diabetes and arteriosclerosis. Based on the strength of this process, mediators produced in the inflammatory site can accomplish the circulation and results in fever (Kassuya *et al.*, 2009). The complex pathophysiological process of inflammation was interceded by numerous signaling molecules, which can be generated from macrophages, leukocytes and mast cells that respond to phagocytic uptake and production of inflammatory mediators (Yu *et al.*, 2010b). The inflammatory mediators including nitric oxide, prostaglandin E2 and tumour necrosis factor that forms edema and results in fluid and proteins extravasations of fluid and proteins and accretion of leucocytes on inflammatory site (White, 1999). Moreover, the cytokines are formed by the immune or central nervous system of cells may directly sensitize the marginal nociceptors (Obreja *et al.*, 2002). Inflammation causes various degenerative diseases including gouty arthritis, rheumatoid arthritis, polymyalgia rheumatic, shoulder tendonitis, heart disease, inflammatory bowel disease and asthma (Iwalewa *et al.*, 2007).

The inflammatory process was divides into two phases namely acute and chronic responses. In acute inflammation, increases of vascular permeability and cellular infiltration to oedema formation, which results in fluid and protein extravasations on inflammatory sites, occur in a short period (Posadas *et al.*, 2004). Chronic inflammation is caused at the time of insufficient acute response which removes the pro-inflammatory agents. Chronic inflammation contains the proliferation of fibroblasts and infiltration of neutrophils along with exudation of fluid. Chronic inflammation may also take place by the perseverance of infection or antigen, tissue injury or poor endogenous anti-inflammatory mechanisms. The macrophages are capable of managing various immunopathological phenomena such as an extra generation of proinflammatory cytokines and inflammatory mediators, which is produced by active iNOS and COX-2 (Walsh, 2003).

Many Non-steroidal anti-inflammatory drugs (NSAIDs) are available to reduce inflammation or swelling by binding to corticoid receptors. These NSAIDs are carboxylic acid-containing drugs namely aspirin, indomethacin, ibuprofen, ketoprofen, flurbiprofen and diclofenac. These synthetic chemical drugs perform in enzyme active sites preventing access of arachidonic acid and terminates cyclooxygenase pathway (Marnett, 2009; Inotai *et al.*, 2010). Regrettably, many researchers reported that NSAIDs have a risk of serious cardiovascular events and severe life-threatening gastrointestinal events (Layton *et al.*, 2008). Moreover, NSAIDs like diclofenac may cause side effects including gastrointestinal disorders when administered by oral route and cutaneous lesions by intramuscular injection and also results in hepatotoxicity (Aydin *et al.*, 2003; Suwalsky *et al.*, 2009). Over the last few decades, plant-based drugs and plant oils play a vital role in the reduction of inflammation. Hence, ethanolpharmacology and drug discovery using natural products have remained an important issue in the current target-rich, lead-poor scenario of pharmaceutical research (Selvum and Jachak, 2004; Shaikh *et al.*, 2015).

1.7 ABOUT CANCER

Cancer is a deadly disease, which causes morbidity and mortality in millions of people around the world. The cancer cells can start, multiply, lodge and grow in various tissues and organs throughout the body, in men there are five most important cancers are lung cancer, prostate cancer, colorectal cancer, stomach cancer and liver cancer, whereas in women breast cancer, colorectal cancer, lung cancer, cervical cancer and stomach cancer (Torre *et al.*, 2015). The oncogenes and tumor suppressor genes are two important key factors in the molecular basis of cancer cell development among differentiated normal cells (Levine and Puzio-Kuter, 2010; Ngo *et al.*, 2015). The activation of oncogenes and inactivation of tumor suppressor genes by naturally occurring gene, which can trigger uncontrolled cell growth and cell proliferation concluded with alteration of cells obtaining carcinogenesis properties (Vander Heiden *et al.*, 2009; Jones and Thompson, 2009; Ward and Thompson 2012). The molecular mechanisms known are underlying cancer development has led to the expansion of a huge number of anticancer drugs.

1.8 CERVICAL CANCER

Cervical cancer is the term for malignant neoplasm arising from cells originating from the cervix uteri (Katrin Sak, 2014; Jin *et al.*, 2014). Cervical cancer is the fourth most common cancer in women with 5,70,000 new cases in 2018 and representing 6.6% of all female cancers. There are roughly 90% of deaths from cervical cancer reported to occur in low- and middle-income countries. There are 7.5% of female cancer deaths is occurred by gynecologic malignancy and the most frequent cause of gynecologic cancer deaths (Muthusami *et al.*, 2013; Garcia *et al.*, 2014). Universally, the increasing mortality rate of cervical cancer was controlled by prevention, early diagnosis, effective screening and treatment programs. There are currently vaccines that protect against common cancer-causing types of human papilloma virus and can significantly reduce the risk of cervical cancer (WHO, 2018). The incidence and mortality of cervical cancer were reduced in developed countries, meanwhile, 80% of new cases take place in the developing countries (Zou *et al.*, 2010). Cervical cancer is generally curable by early detection, but the treatment of metastatic or recurrent carcinoma is lack of effective with severe side effects (Muthusami *et al.*, 2013). Therapies like surgery, radiotherapy, chemotherapy and immunotherapy are used to kill the cancer cells (Chen *et al.*, 2013). Radiotherapy is used to the majority of patients with early-stage cervical cancer. The chemotherapy is used for advanced-stage patients in which the prognosis remains very poor (Zhu *et al.*, 2013). Both therapies as chemotherapy and radiotherapy can cause severe lethality on normal cells and result in toxicity (Singh *et al.*, 2013).

At this Juncture, there is a necessity to reduce the cervical cancer morbidity rate and mortality rate by developing more effective and less toxic anticancer agents with novel therapeutic intervention strategies (Katrin Sak, 2014). As per the earlier reports, there are several effective anticancer drugs are isolated from plant sources (Kitdamrongtham *et al.*, 2013). In the last few decades, the plants have an extensive approach on potential antitumor activity with modern anticancer drugs such as vincristine, camptothecin, vinblastine, taxol, adriamycin, paclitaxel and etoposide (Krifa *et al.*, 2013). There are numerous unexploited resources still remained in herbal medicines, hence the researchers searching new promising leads from plants against cancer to the development of novel chemotherapeutics (Ju *et al.*, 2012; Alonso-Castro *et al.*, 2013).

1.9 SCOPE OF THE PRESENT STUDY

Therefore, it is anticipated that plants can provide potential bioactive compounds for the development of new molecules to combat cancer diseases. Based on the above scientific and technological information, the present study is undertaken to investigate the effect of biologically active compounds isolated from promising medicinal plants selected from the Thiruvadisoolam forest of Kanchipuram District of Tamil Nadu for antioxidant properties include anti-inflammatory and anticancer activity. The current study would be helpful to develop a new plant based drugs, from any of the selected plant species, which may be potential in above pharmacological activities. The methanolic crude plant extracts enriched with anti-cancer compounds and activity would be further purified for the isolation of bioactive anti-cancerous compounds. After the isolation and characterization of bio active compounds, it will be studied for all the molecular targets responsible for cancer studies. Further, the chemical analogs would be synthesized for all the identified anti-cancerous compounds, which may be useful for commercial preparation of drugs for combating this deadly disease after conducting sufficient clinical trials.

1.10 OBJECTIVES

The present study was aimed at the following objectives:

- ✓ To conduct an ethnobotanical survey of Thiruvadisoolam forest, Kanchipuram District, Tamil Nadu, India.
- ✓ The qualitative and quantitative profiles of phytochemical constituents from selected medicinal plants from above survey to be analysed.
- ✓ To assess the antimicrobial activity of Phyto-constituents isolated from the above-selected plant species.
- ✓ To ascertain an antioxidant activity by 1, 1-Diphenyl-2-picryl-hydroxyl free radical method (DPPH), Phosphomolybdenum assay, Fe^{3+} Reducing power assay of crude extracts of above-selected plants species.
- ✓ Study of the Phyto-anatomical structures of the potential plant *C. albidum*. Leaf and Petiole.
- ✓ Isolation and purification of potential bioactive compounds from *C. albidum* by TLC and column chromatography.
- ✓ Characterization and molecular identification of isolated and purified biocompounds from *C. albidum*.

CHAPTER- II

REVIEW OF LITERATURE

2.1 TRADITIONAL SYSTEM OF MEDICINE IN INDIA

India owns its traditional system of medicine such as Ayurveda, Siddha and Unani. Those medical systems originate in the ancient Vedas and other scriptures. The Ayurveda concept appeared and developed between 2500 and 500 BC in India. India is a developing country, which contains tremendous storage of medicinal plants that are used in various traditional medical treatments. In the traditional medicine system, alternative drugs are obtained from herbs, minerals and organic matter, whereas medicinal plants are used only in herbal drugs (Pandey *et al.*, 2013). In worldwide, 60 percent of people preferring alternative medicines, which are not only used by developing countries but also used in developed countries wherever those modern medicines dominate (Ballabh and Caucasia, 2007).

The classical transcripts of Indian traditional medicine system as Ayurveda include Rigveda, Atharvaveda, Charaka Samhita and Sushruta Samhita (Ravishankar and Shukla 2007). Ajeet (2018), reported that India has registered 2,50,000 medical practitioners of Ayurvedic system and 7,00,000 in modern medicine. Almost 20,000 medicinal plants have been documented but traditional practitioners exercised only 7,000–7,500 plants for various remedies. The sum of medicinal plants used in various medicinal systems include Ayurveda 2000, folk 4500, Homeopathy 800, Siddha 1300, Tibetan 500, Unani 1000 and Modern medicine 200 (Pandey *et al.*, 2013).

2.2 IMPORTANCE OF ETHNOBOTANICAL STUDY

Medicinal plants play a key role in human health care not only in medicine but also used as food. About 80% of the world's population relies on the use of traditional medicine, which is predominately based on plant materials. The traditional medicine refers to a board range of ancient, natural Health care practices including folk/tribal practices as well as Ayurveda, Siddha and Unani (Thamizhvanan *et al.*, 2017). Chanchal *et al.* (2017) have studied *Carissa carandas* (L.) is a medicinal plant belonging to the Apocynaceae family and it is represented about 89 species in India. Many plants of this family are the sources of important constituents of therapeutic importance. It naturally grows in the Himalayas at a height of 300 to 1800 meters in the Siwalik Hills from sea level and requires full exposure to sun and unfavorable to humidity. Out of the 8 Indian species, three are of economically important and good medicinal values. Sangeeta Devi *et al.*, (2017) has studied *Euphorbia's heart* belongs to the family *Euphorbiaceae*. It is a small annual herb and grows up to a height of 40 cm which is used in the treatment of many diseases including bronchitis, skin diseases, cough, hay asthma, bowel disease, worm infestation, kidney stones, bronchial disease, sedative, anxiolytic, analgesic and antipyretic.

Maribeth Laurente *et al.* (2017) have studied the use of plants as a source of herbal therapeutic agents that have been established long before modernization has completely conquered earth. The Philippines is known for its rich biodiversity, especially in its flora. The antimicrobial, antioxidant, and anti-inflammatory activity of the selected plant materials can be correlated with their phytochemistry. Sankaraiah *et al.* (2017) investigated the flowers of *C. auriculata* Linn. that are used for various conditions of ailments in traditional systems of medicine since ancient times. Phytochemical and physicochemical analysis of powdered drugs proved to be useful for various healthcare system that differentiate the powdered drug material, in which the High-performance thin-layer chromatography (HPTLC) analysis showed the presence of important phytoconstituents.

The research report on *C. carandus* summarized that it has many uses as it is used in traditional medicine, and modern medical research has found that it has many beneficial properties. Its leaves feed the tussah silkworm; the wood is used for making household utensils, such as large cooking spoons, and the root can be pounded to a paste to make insect repellant. The plant is also an alternative source of oil, hydrocarbon, and phytochemicals (Rajaram *et al.*, 2013). Sami Ashgar (2017) evaluated medicinal plants that acquired great attention for their miracle properties against various human illnesses. Venkata Kullai Setty *et al.* (2011) analyzed the herbs are plants, that are used in a number of ways including cooking, religious, rituals and medicines. In botany, herbs are defined as seed-producing plants with non-woody stems that wither and die back to the ground after season growth. Mohamed Saleem Gani and Nalini Devi (2015) reported that *Euphorbia prostrata* is used traditionally in the Ayurveda system of medicine in India for the treatment of liver diseases and also used as a liver tonic. Bhargava *et al.* (2012) determined the *Zingiber Officinale* is a common condiment for various foods and beverages and a long history of the important traditional medicinal herb for the treatment of stomach disorders. The constituents present in ginger have potent antioxidant and anti-inflammatory activities.

Bokhad and Rothe (2012) stated that day by day faith of people on herbal medicine increased due to the side effect of synthetic drugs and people hence started looking back to the traditional knowledge of plants for their health care system. Certain local practitioners and traditional healers use the decoction of the fruit of *Combretum albidum* (G. Don) in the treatment of diarrhea and dysentery, stem barks used in jaundice. Therefore, the present study deals with the preliminary phytochemical analysis of stem, leaf, flower and fruit using six different solvent extracts. It helps with the scientific documentation and standardization of raw plant material used in medicine and its worldwide acceptance. Manjula and Selvin Jebaraj Norman (2017) reported that the medicinal plants occupy a very important place throughout the world, due to its significance of human health. There are multi-potential plants like *Phyllanthus reticulatus* which has the capacity to cure many ailments. The tribal community Malasar of Nilgiri Biosphere is efficient healers and they use this plant to cure any ailments. Malasars is a highly respectable tribe in this locality, owing to the traditional knowledge they possess about the medicinal values of specific plants grown in their ecosystem. The investigation of Rajmohan and Sumithra (2017), prove the potentially toxic medicinal plants and mineral drugs have an important role in Siddha medicine preparation. Since these drugs produce side effects on humans, their toxic principles found to be reduced for use in medicines.

2.3 NATURAL PRODUCTS FROM PLANTS

Plants have a tremendous source of natural products which are used as food and medicine for human and animals. The consumption of the plants and their products for nutritional value and traditional medicine or complementary medicine were reported by Jonas *et al.* (2013). Anthocyanin is the natural pigment that can easily be extracted from plants especially *Carissa carandus* Linn. which contains a large amount of natural anthocyanin. The anthocyanin has significant antioxidant activity and it is a Thai traditional fermented pork sausage called Nham (Sueprasarn *et al.*, 2017).

Curcumin (1E,6E)-1,7-bis(4-hydroxy-3-methoxyphenyl)hepta-1,6-diene-3,5-dione, also known as diferuloyl methane, is the main ingredient of *Curcuma longa*, which is yellow in color and represents a lipophilic polyphenol and has an effective role on anti-inflammatory, antioxidant, anticancer and antimicrobial activities (Epstein *et al.*, 2010). Colchicine is a troponin derivative, which is the most important alkaloid of *Colchicum autumnal* and used against gout attacks. Moreover, the US FDA approved colchicine for the treatment and prevention of familial Mediterranean fever and acute gout flares (Stanton *et al.*, 2011). Resveratrol is a stilbene derivative 5-[(E)-2-(4-hydroxyphenyl) ethenyl] benzene-1,3-diol, major phytoalexin and it is presented in various plants and dietary products including grapevines, red wines and peanuts (Gescher *et al.*, 2013). Capsaicin is a hydrophobic alkaloid (E)-N-[(4-hydroxy-3- methoxyphenyl) methyl]-8-methylnon-6-enamide, present in chili peppers (Solanaceae) and is accountable for the classic spiciness of the fruits of Capsicum. Capsaicin is used as remedies to relieve the pain of muscles and joints, neuropathic pain in non-diabetic adults and neuropathic pain related with postherpetic neuralgia (Caterina *et al.*, 1997; O'Neill, *et al.*, 2012; Haanpaa and Treede, 2012).

Epigallocatechin-3-gallate (EGCG) is an polyphenol compound, [(2R,3R)-5,7-dihydroxy-2-(3,4,5-trihydroxyphenyl)-3,4-dihydro-2H-chromen-3-yl]3,4,5-trihydroxybenzoate, usually found in *Camellia sinensis* that contains various biological properties like antioxidant, anticancer, anti-inflammatory, anti-infective, antiangiogenetic as well as chemopreventive effects (Singh *et al.*, 2011; Furst and Zundorf, 2014). Quercetin is a flavonol comes under a group of flavonoid compounds 2-(3,4-dihydroxyphenyl)-3,5,7-trihydroxychromen-4-one. Quercetin is found in grapevines, apples, berries, red onions, broccoli, and capers. This compound contains a broad spectrum of biological activity like anti-inflammatory, anti-infectious, antioxidant, anticancer, neuroprotective, antihypertensive and reducing blood glucose level (Hirpara, *et al.*, 2009, Bischoff, 2008; Chirumbolo, 2010; Larson *et al.*, 2012). The molecular structure of curcumin, epigallocatechin-3-gallate, capsaicin, quercitin, colchicine and revestrol were presented in **Figure** 1.for reference.

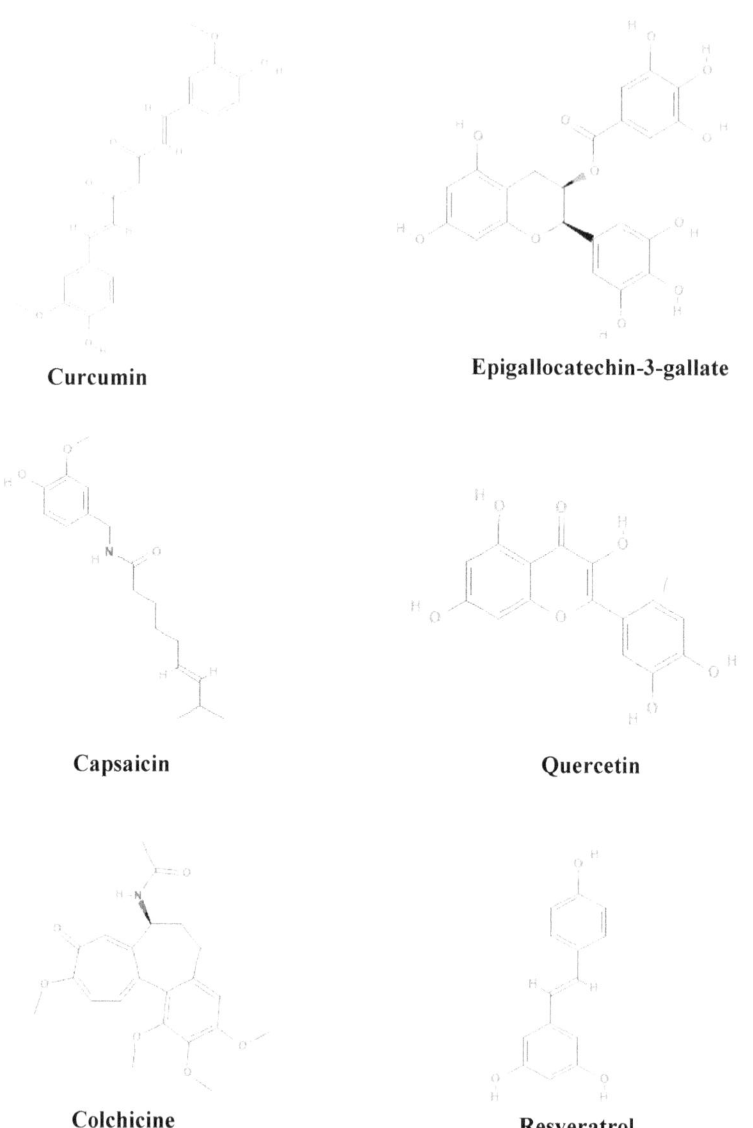

FIGURE 1: The Molecular Structure of Curcumin, Epigallocatechin-3-Gallate, Capsaicin, Quercitin, Colchicine and Revestrol

2.4 METABOLIC COMPOUNDS OF PLANTS

Ashvin and co-workers (2012) isolated 19 phytochemicals from ethanolic extracts of roots of *Carissa carandus* Linn. which are useful for the development and growth of the plant. The phytochemicals estimation is screened by using three different solvents such as ethanol, chloroform and aqueous. The wild and edible fruits such as *Coccinia indica, C. carandas* and *Ficus benghalensis,* which contains alkaloids, flavonoids, steroids, phenols, and saponins (Anand *et al.,* 2017). Gouri Dhar *et al.* (2017) have investigated that solvents affect the extraction of phenolic and flavonoid substances and the antioxidant activity of fruit extract of *A. chaplasha* and *C. carandas.* In this study, the phenolic content and antioxidant activity were found to highest in 70% acetone extract and lowest in 100% acetone extract whilst flavonoid content was highest in pure ethanol extracts of both fruit. A strong correlation was found between the phenolic contents and antioxidant activities. Venkata Pavan Kumar *et al.* (2016) evaluated the cardiotonic activity of aqueous extract of the whole plant of *Carmona retusa* (Vahl) Masam. Phytochemical screening of whole plant material revealed that the major constituent of *C. retusa* was phenols. Further, the cardiotonic effect of aqueous extract of the whole plant of *C. retusa* was studied by using isolated frog heart perfusion technique (IFHP) in which calcium free ringer solution was used as a vehicle for administration of aqueous extract of *C. retusa* as a test extract and digoxin as a standard.

Monisha *et al.* (2017) investigated that the phytochemical studies of leaves and pods of *Cassia auriculata* and found the biological activity. Since it has antimicrobial, antioxidant, anti-inflammatory properties, aqueous and methanol extracts were used to identify the medicinal properties of *C. auriculata* and the chromatography studies of leaves and pods have been described. Shammi *et al.* (2018) studied the petroleum ether, ethyl acetate, and methanol extracts of *Phyllanthus reticulatus.* Poir. (Euphorbiaceae) and were chosen for pharmacological screening. The analgesic activity of the extracts was performed using acetic acid-induced writhing in mice and Formalin induced to have an analgesic activity of the dose 100 and 200mg/kg body weight in the tested models compared to control. So, methanolic extract of *Phyllanthus meticulous* and *Mimosa pigra* has remarkable Analgesic and Anti-inflammatory activities. Achinta Saha *et al.* (2007) have studied the petroleum ether, ethyl acetate, and methanol extracts of *Phyllanthus reticulatus* Poir. (Euphorbiaceae) which were chosen for pharmacological screening. In the acetic acid-induced writhing test, the ethyl acetate extract in doses of 150 and 300 mg=kg showed 51.23 and 65.12% inhibition of writhing, respectively.

Various phytochemical compounds of leaf extracts of *C. carandas* and their antioxidant properties, antimicrobial activities and cytotoxic potentials were studied by Bint-e-Sadek *et al.* (2013). Akansha and Gursimran (2015), found that *C. carandas* has encloses major bioactive constituents, which impart medicinal value to the herb, are alkaloids, flavonoids, saponins and large amounts of cardiac glycosides, triterpenoids, phenolic compounds, and tannins. Sangeeta Devi and co-workers (2017), found phytochemical components such as alkaloids, flavonoids, terpenoids, glycoside, saponin, tannins, carbohydrates and amino acid were present in the methanolic extract of *Euphorbia hirta*. The phytochemical screening of *E. hirta* was studied and found that revealed that the plant contained reducing sugars, terpenoids, alkaloids, steroids, tannins, proteins, fats, oils, gums, mucilages, glycoside, saponin, coumarin, cardiac glycosides, anthraquinones, flavonoids, and phenolic compounds (Ali Esmail Al-Snafi, 2017). Venumadhav and Seshagirirao (2017), have conducted the study to screen the phytochemical compounds present in the phylloclade of *Euphorbia caducifolia* and found the extracts with total phenolic and flavonoid content and antioxidant activities. Carbohydrates, phenols, flavonoids, tannins, glycosides in water extract and terpenoids along with phenols and flavonoids in methanol, whereas hexane contains a maximum of terpenoids and reducing sugars.

The phytochemical screening, proximate analysis, mineral elements and antinutritional composition of *Zingiber officinale* rhizome were carried out by Osabor *et al.* (2015), with a view to assessing its nutritional and medicinal values. The Phytochemical screening revealed that *Z. officinale* has good secondary plant metabolites which justify its therapeutic utility. Bhargava *et al.*, (2012) observed that *Z. Officinale* extract has phytochemicals of alkaloids, saponins, tannins, flavonoids, terpenoid, and phlorotannin. Rajkumar *et al.* (2017) investigated the antioxidant-rich phytochemicals such as alkaloids, phenols, flavonoids, tannins, saponins, terpenoids, steroids, carbohydrates, glycosides, amino acids and proteins in the different solvent extracts of *Carmona retusa* (Vahl) Masamune leaves. Ida Christi *et al.* (2017) evaluated the phytochemical nature of the plant *Cassia auriculata* Linn. and comparatively study the antidiabetic activity of ethanolic extract and fresh juice of flower in diabetic rats. The flowers are quantitatively evaluated for phytochemical analysis like flavonoid content, total phenol content, etc. and documented. Further, the methanolic extract and fresh juice of the flowers were screened for their protective effect towards the reduction in blood sugar level in albino rats by hypoglycemic activity in normal rats and OGTT methods.

Sachin and Amit (2014) determined the phytochemicals of petroleum ether, methanol and chloroform extracts of *Cassia auriculata* leaves which shows anthelmintic activity against earthworms due to the presence of alkaloids, tannins flavonoids, glycosides, saponins along with proteins. Manipal *et al.* (2017) reported that the flavonoids in barks of selected taxa of *Combretaceae* viz. *Terminalia* (*Terminalia alata, Terminalia arjuna, Terminalia bellirica, Terminalia catappa, Terminalia chebula, Terminalia pallida, Terminalia paniculata), Anogeissus acuminate, Anogeissus latifolia, Calycopteris floribunda, Combretum albidum* and *Quisqualis indica*. They conclude that all the selected taxa Barks of *Combretaceae* possess and can be regarded as promising candidates for natural plant sources which contain high value dietary rich flavonoids.

The investigation of Florence and Regini Balasingh (2016a), on bioactive components present in the leaf extracts of *Gmelina asiatica* showed the presence of bioactive components such as alkaloids, carbohydrates, glycosides, coumarins, quinones, saponins, steroids, terpenoids, proteins, phytosterols, tannins, and flavonoids. Neelam *et al.* (2017) made study on phytochemical analysis and antioxidant properties of *Brassica oleracea* (fluorescence), *Terminalia chebula* (fruits), *Terminalia belerica* (fruits), *Phyllanthus Emblica* (fruits) *Abutilon Indicum* (stems and leaves) and *Swertia chirata* (stems). The aqueous, as well as ethanolic extracts of these selected plant materials showed the presence of different phytochemicals *i.e.* alkaloids, phenolic compounds, protein, saponins, carbohydrate, and glycosides. Sudhira *et al.* (2015) reported that the phytochemicals such as flavonoids, steroids, tannins, alkaloids, glycosides, phenols and reducing sugars have capable of scavenging the free radicals.

2.5 PHARMOCOGNOSTIC STUDY

Pharmacognosy deals with the standardization and authentication of natural drugs obtained from various natural sources, especially plants. Many researchers have been doing research on pharmacognosy to identifying notorious plant species and authentication of traditional medicinal plants with the help of morphological, physicochemical and phytochemical analysis. Sumitra (2014) reviewed and discussed the requirement and importance of pharmacognostic study over the medicinal plants and the study deals with the important parameters to standardize and authenticate the medicinal plants, hence through the adulteration and substitution can be prevented.

The parameters including in pharmacognostic studies such as macroscopic study, organoleptic characters, microscopic study, fluorescence analysis, textural study, phytochemical analysis and physicochemical analysis (ash values, moisture content, loss on drying, extractive values) are enlisted along with their importance. Florence and Regini Balasingh (2016a), investigated to provide the information on the anatomical features of the leaves and stems of the plant *Gmelina asiatica*. Leaf and stem anatomy of *G. asiatica* was undertaken by rotary microtome and examined on photomicrographs. Anatomical characters such as echinate epidermal cells, glandular trichomes, anomocytic stomata, calcium oxalate crystals, periderm cylinder, phellem cells and vascular bundle of leaf and stem explain typical features of Verbenaceae.

2.6 ANTIMICROBIAL PROPERTIES OF PLANTS

Many research investigations by various scientists worldwide on the antimicrobial activity such as antibacterial and antifungal activity of enormous plant species were reported to found significant results and the potential of the plants. Waseem *et al*., (2017) reported that antimicrobial effect of *E. hirta* plant extract which has potential activity against *Proteus mirabilis, Listeria monocytogenes, Clostridium absonum, Aspergillus niger, Aspergillus fumigates* and *Arthrographis cuboidal.* It was concluded that their effective antimicrobial property was due to be the presence of alkaloid, flavonoid, saponin, terpenoid, steroid, and sterols. Savita and Pushpa (2017) also studied the aerial parts of *E. hirta* and resulted that the plant extracts showed a wide spectrum of inhibition against the test pathogens thus justifying the use of the plant in traditional medicine. Muhammad *et al.* (2017), investigated the phytochemical content as well as antimicrobial properties of Nigerian and Indian ginger and were assessed in an effort to compare and validate the medicinal potential of the plant. Aqueous, solvent and hydroethanolic extracts of Indian and Nigerian ginger prepared by the solvent extraction process were found to contain a high amount of secondary metabolites. Riaz *et al.* (2015) performed the phytochemical evaluation and an antimicrobial assay of ginger root extract which were available in the local farms of Lahore. The study on ginger possesses a noticeable antimicrobial activity which was confirmed by checking the susceptibility of different strains of bacteria and fungi by measuring the zone of inhibition. Kaushik and Goyal (2011) revealed that the pattern of inhibition of microorganism varied with the solvent used for extraction of plant species and the organism tested. Plant extracts prepared in organic solvents provided more consistent antibacterial activity as compared to aqueous extracts. The methanol extract was the most active against the maximum number of bacterial species tested and found effective on Gram-positive bacteria which were sensitive as compared to Gram-negative bacteria according to various studies.

Syed *et al.* (2017) have studied the antimicrobial activities of medicinal plants such as *Jasminum grandiflorum* L., *Spinacia oleracea* L., *Coriandrum sativum* L., *and Zingiber officinale* Roscoe. The antibacterial activity of the methanolic extracts of these plants was tested against 12 Gram-positive and 18 Gram-negative bacteria at 1000 µg/disc concentration by the disc diffusion method which shows the methanolic extracts of leaves of *J. grandiflorum* and *S. oleracea* showed significant antibacterial activity. Raja *et al.* (2013) have studied the antimicrobial activity of aerial parts of chloroform extract of *C. auriculata* L. shown antimicrobial activity against 2 gram-positive and 2 gram-negative human pathogenic bacteria and few species of fungi.

Sami Ashgar (2017) evaluated antibacterial effectiveness of *Curcuma longa* and *Z. officinale* (Ginger) extracted with aqueous, 70% ethanol and ethyl acetate solvents against 13 American type cultures collection (ATCC) strains by minimum inhibitory concentration (MIC) and minimum bactericidal concentration (MBC) assay. The results show that the extracts exhibited moderate to significant antibacterial activity. Chandrappa *et al.* (2012) investigated on *Carmona retusa* leaf extracted with petroleum ether, methanol and chloroform separately and tested for antibacterial activity against four bacteria using the agar diffusion method. The experimental data indicated that all extracts exhibit moderate to appreciable antibacterial activities against *Bacillus subtilis, Klebsiella pneumonia, Shigella flexneri,* and *Pseudomonas aeruginosa.*

Methanol, chloroform and aqueous extracts of *Cassia auriculata* leaf were subjected for antimicrobial activity by well -diffusion method against 6 bacterial strains namely *Bacillus cereus, Staphylococcus aureus, Escherichia coli, Klebsiella pneumonia, Pseudomonas aeruginosa,* and *Proteus mirabilis* by Murugan *et al.* (2013) and found effective antibacterial activity. Antibacterial activity on C. *albidum* was studied by disk diffusion assay against seven bacterial strains and found lower antimicrobial activities were recorded by the leaf and bark extracts of C. *albidum* (Arundhati Das *et al.*, 2018). Florence and Regini Balasingh (2016b) investigated that the *in-vitro* antibacterial activities of the crude extracts and essential oil extracted from *Gmelina asiatica* leaf for the control of human pathogenic bacteria such as *Actinomyces howelli, Bacillus circulans, Staphylococcus aureus, Streptococcus pyogenes Escherichia coli, Pseudomonas aeruginos*a and *Proteus Vulgaris*. All the crude extracts have moderate activity against all the tested pathogens and the essential oils had very less antibacterial activity against *Actinomyces, Bacillus* and *Proteus* when compared with standard antibiotic kanamycin. Glad Mohesh *et al.* (2015) reported that the methanolic extract of *Strychnos nux vomica* flowers was able to inhibit all the microorganisms chosen however its effect was higher with *Candida albicans* and *Klebsiella pneumonia* in which the Chloramphenicol (10ug/ml) was the standard drug of choice.

2.7 ANTIOXIDANT POTENTIAL OF MEDICINAL PLANTS

Vitamin C or ascorbic acid is known by its electron-donating ability, thanks to which it prevents the accumulation of oxidizing agents and free radicals in the cells and tissues. Some studies have shown that the intake of this compound can inhibit disease progression in the lung, cervix, breast, stomach, liver, and colon cancer (Singh *et al.*, 2011). The reduction in the number of DPPH molecules can be correlated with the number of available hydroxyl (-OH) groups. The antioxidant activities of the chloroform, ethanolic fruit and root extracts of *C. carandus* may be probably due to the presence of compounds with hydroxyl groups (Chanchal *et al.*, 2017). Muhammad *et al.* (2017) have studied that the phytochemical content and antioxidant potential of Nigerian and Indian ginger were assessed in an effort to compare and validate the medicinal potential of the plant. Rajkumar *et al.* (2017) investigated the phytochemical screening and *in- vitro* free radical scavenging ability of the different solvent extracts of *Carmona retusa* (Vahl) Masamune leaves.

Rupam Bharti *et al.* (2012) reviewed and summarized that the natural antioxidants from plant sources are capable to scavenge toxic free radicals from the complex biological system. Antioxidants applying their mode of action by repressing the development of ROS or enzyme inhibition or through chelating trace elements. The presence of antioxidants in different plant parts including phenolic compounds, ascorbic acid and vitamin E have the capability to diminish the oxidative damage, which influences various diseases like atherosclerosis, cancer, arthritis, cardiovascular diseases, cataracts, immune deficiency diseases, ageing, and diabetes.

The antioxidant activity of phenolic compounds from traditional Chinese medicinal plants was studied by Cai *et al.* (2004) which is related to anticancer properties, encompasses 112 species from 50 plant families. Moreover, there is a positive and significant linear relationship between total phenol content and antioxidant activity was reported by several authors. Major types of phenolic compounds such as flavonoids, phenolic acids, tannins, lignans, stilbenes, coumarins, quinones and curcuminoids are having the antioxidant properties. These substances are presented in common vegetables and fruits, which exhibited stronger antioxidant activity. Pourmorad *et al.* (2006) concluded that the Iranian medicinal plants especially, *Mellilotus officinalis* have a large amount of flavonoid and phenolic compounds. These compounds possess significant antioxidant activity due to the presence of hydroxyl groups in phenolic compounds and their chemical structure. The statement of Esmaeili and Sonboli (2010), the DPPH is broadly using compound to estimate the antioxidant activity of foods or plants and also to quantify antioxidants in complex biological systems.

Abhishek *et al.* (2013) showed interest for finding safe and suitable antioxidants of plant source. They have screened around 35 plants, among them antioxidant-rich four plants such as *Acacia catechu, Holopetelea integrifolia, Adenanthera pavonia,* and *Terminalia paniculata* were recorded. The phytoconstituents of selected medicinal plants were correlated with the antioxidant properties. Srinivasan (2014) declared that the spices involving in free radical scavenging activity, development of antioxidant components in tissues, mammalian system and suppression of lipid peroxidase. The antioxidant activity of the compounds from this spice involves only single or more than one process from, free radical scavenging activity, improving the antioxidant molecules in tissues, LPO suppression, decreasing the induction of nitric oxide synthase activity, stimulating the endogenous antioxidant enzyme action and reduction of arachidonate related 2-cyclooxygenase and 5-lipoxygenase enzymes. Srinivasan (2017) accounted that the rhizome of *Z. officinale* which is used as a spice in food and drinks due to their pungency and piquant flavor. Moreover, this rhizome is extensively used in ayurvedic,

Chinese and Unani medicines for several remedies including inflammation, pain, and gastrointestinal disorders.

Narayanaswamy and Balkrishnan (2011) investigated the total phenolic content and antioxidant properties of 13 important medicinal plants such as *Alpina calcarata, Ocimum basillicum, Jatropa curcas, Acorus calamus, Verbascum thapsus, Jatropa gossipifolia, Jatropa multifida, Strebilis aspera, Hyptis suaveolens, Solanum indicum, Clitorria ternate, Passiflora edulis* and *Sauropus androgynous*. The DPPH scavenging potential of the aqueous extracts and ethanolic extracts of above plants was tested and reported that *H. suaveolens* showed highest inhibition of DPPH radical. Moreover their findings exposed that hydrogen donating ability of phenolics may the reason for potential radical scavenging activity of above medicinal plants. The antioxidant potential of different plant species have been thoroughly studied by various authors including Elumalai and Kasinathan (2016); Mardani-Talaee *et al.* (2016). Firdose Kolar *et al.* (2017) have studied the antioxidant activity of aqueous and ethanol extracts of four plants from the genus *Cassia* which was evaluated by various antioxidant assays, including ferric reducing antioxidant power (FRAP), DPPH free radical scavenging, metal chelating activity, phosphomolybdenum reducing power, hydrogen peroxide radical scavenging, hydroxyl radical scavenging, deoxyribose degradation, and β-carotene bleaching assay. The possible antioxidant mechanism of the ethanol extract can be due to its hydrogen or electron-donating and direct free radical scavenging properties. Irsa Tahir *et al.* (2016) have studied the antioxidant potential of a methanol extract of *Phyllanthus Emblica* leaves (PELE) which was determined by *in vitro* methods as well as by an *in vivo* animal model, along with HPLC-DAD screening for Phyto-constituents.

Vijayanand and Sanjana (2017) studied the phytoconstituents of *Phyllanthus emblica, Ananas comosus* and *Momordica charantia* extracts for its antioxidant activity and its potential as a preservative. The antioxidant effects were evaluated for radical scavenging activity using FRAP with certain modifications and found the chloroform extract of *M. charantia* revealed highest free radical scavenging activity. Similarly, the ethanolic extracts of *P. emblica* have also possess significant scavenging effect. Total phenolic content of the extracts *P. emblica, Ananas comosus, M. charantia* were determined by the Follin Ciocaltea method in which positive correlations were found between the total phenolic content of the extracts and antioxidant activity.

The terpenoids have been found to possess antioxidant and antimicrobial properties which was reported by several scientists (Singh and Singh, 2003). The presence of phenols in the extract may explain its potent bioactivities as tannins are known to possess potent antioxidants (Pereira *et al.*, 2007 and Gulumser *et al.*, 2010). The investigation has shown that the methanol extract dosage active phytochemicals (terpenoids, flavonoids, coumarins, and phenols) are able to show antioxidants. The strong antioxidant activity was confirmed in methanol extract. Possibly it will be due to the strong occurrence of a polyphenolic compound such as terpenoids and phenols. These findings provide scientific evidence to support uses and indicate a promising potential for the development of antimicrobial and antioxidant drugs from *C. albidum.*

Tannins are the enormous groups of phenolic compounds used as medicinal agents in a number of diseases like rhinorrhea, leucorrhoea, and diarrhea. Saponins are essential phytochemicals as they are found to have a hypolipidemic, antidiabetic and anticancer activity which was present in a noticeable amount in the plant extracts of various medically important plant species.

However, hydroxyl radical is more reactive in the induction of lesions in cellular molecules whilst hydrogen peroxide is sufficiently able to cross the nuclear membrane and cause damage to the DNA molecule. Therefore, effective and safe antioxidants acquired sustainably from biodiversity, which can diminish the threat of free radicals and reactive oxygen species damage over generation (Lopes *et al.*, 2013). It is observed that from various scientific reports as the phenolic compounds exhibit their antioxidant activity by various mechanisms such as donation of hydrogen atoms to free radicals and through connection to change metal ions resulting in more stable forms (Kumar *et al.*, 2014; Floegel *et al.*, 2011; Mehta *et al.*, 2013).

Since the plants exposed promising antioxidant activity, it requires advance studies to throw light on their chemical composition and antioxidant properties (Elumalai and Kasinathan, 2016). Many oxidative stress related diseases are gaining importance as a result of the accumulation of free radicals in the body. A number of researches are going on global aimed towards finding natural antioxidants of plant origins to solve the issues of human cellular disorders. Therefore, it is observed that from the present investigation on the methanolic extract of *C. albidum* is a possible source of natural antioxidants and this can be acceptable for its uses in folkloric medicines. Renuka Chaphalkar *et al.* (2017)

investigated the protective effect of the hydroalcoholic extract of *P. emblica* bark in ethanol-induced hepatotoxicity model in rats. In their study, total phenolics, flavonoid and tannin content and *in vitro* antioxidant activities were determined by using H_2O_2 scavenging and ABTS decolorization assays. The hydroalcholic extract by *p. emblica* mediated hepatoprotection could be due to its free radical scavenging and antioxidant activity that may be ascribed to its antioxidant components namely, ellagic acid and gallic acid.

2.8 ROLE OF MEDICINAL PLANTS IN ANTIINFLAMMATORY ACTIVITY

There is a necessity to develop safety, novel and effective anti-inflammatory drugs instead of NSAIDs to reduce the gastrointestinal side effects.There are most effective and novel anti-inflammatory drugs like Celecoxib, Rofecoxib, and Valdecoxib was withdrawn on the pharmaceutical market due to their major cardio functioning side effects in elderly people, pregnant women and newborn baby (Garcia Rodriguez *et al.*, 2008; Vonkeman and van de Laar, 2010). Drugs produced from the medicinal plants have been the alternatives of NSAID's which acts as a new therapeutic agent. Many researchers proved that phytochemicals like flavonoids, coumarins, terpenoids, saponins, and alkaloids have a major role in inflammation protection (Selvum *et al.*, 2004; Yasser and Nabil, 2012).

Prostaglandins are the end product of lipoxygenase and COX pathways that perform as a secondary messenger and concerned in several immunologic responses. The biosynthesis of Prostaglandins was inhibited by flavonoids of Ajmodadi Churna, which is the extract of 12 ingredients such as fruits of *Trachyspermum Ammi*, *Embelia Ribes*, *Anethum graveolens*, *Piper longum*, *Piper nigrum*, *Terminalia chebula*, wood of *Cedrus deodara*, aerial parts of *Plumbago zeylanica*, stem of *Piper longum*, Root of *Argyreia Nervosa*, Rhizome of *Zingiber officinale* and Rock Salt (Min *et al.*, 2010; Ram *et al.*, 2012), which observed to be boost immune system of human body.

Ojewole (2005) investigated the antinociceptive, anti-inflammatory and antidiabetic properties of aqueous leaf extract of *Bryophyllum pinnatum* in experimental animal models in which anti-inflammatory activity of the extract was determined in fresh egg albumin-induced pedal (paw) edema. The presence of flavonoids, polyphenols, triterpenoids and other chemical constituents in the plant may inhibit the fresh egg albumin-induced acute inflammation. Ilavarasan *et al.* (2005) suggested that the bark extracts of *Cassia fistula* have strong anti-inflammatory activity in the acute and chronic inflammation model in rats due to the presence of flavonoids and bioflavonoids. ROS is most important to cause the pathogenesis of inflammatory diseases.

Julie (2009) reported that curcumin from the Indian spice turmeric *Curcuma longa* possessing a potential anti-inflammatory activity by inhibiting the COX-1 and COX-2 expression activity. Benni *et al.* (2011) studied the effect of *Aegle marmelos* root aqueous extract for anti-inflammatory activity in albino rats using Carrageenan induced paw edema model and cotton pellet induced granuloma and found effective in the experiments. Shaikh *et al.* (2015) evaluated the *in vitro* and *in vivo* anti-inflammatory potential of Indian traditional medication plants such as *Terminalia Billerica*, *Plumbago zeylanica*, *Cissus quadrangularis* and *Terminalia chebula*. The study indicates all the plants inhibit COX-2 activity as compared to COX-1, especially *T. balearica* and *T. chebula* which showed significant COX-2 inhibition and have a potential role in the inhibition of edema formation.

2.9 PLANT-BASED ANTICANCER AGENTS

Cancer is considered as a multifaceted and non-curable disease. Recently, traditional medicines sourced from various plant species have been applied for the treatment of cancers around the world. Many antitumor agents have been reported to induce apoptotic cell death which plays a critical role in killing of tumor cells in cancer therapy (Sakinehsalehi *et al.*, 2016). Cervical cancer is a leading cause of cancer-related deaths in women worldwide (Siegel *et al.*, 2016). Human Papilloma Viruses (HPV) infection is the major risk factor for the prevalence of cervical cancer. Moore *et al.* (2012) considered that HPVs, HPV-16, and HPV18 are responsible for 70% of cervical cancer pathogenesis. Even though, the treatments like chemo-radiotherapy and surgery can cure 80–95% of early-stage cervical cancer. The prevention and treatment of cervical cancer were following by various therapeutic strategies like vaccination and chemotherapeutic drug combinations. However, both vaccinations and chemotherapeutic drugs are toxic when consuming in overdoses. However, plant based natural products have a significant role and gained a lot of attention due to the fewer side effects (Lui *et al.*, 2009).

Researchers from different parts of the world suggested that PTEN/PI3K/AKT/STAT3 signaling pathways are the most important factor to developing cervical carcinogenesis.

The activation of PI3K/AKT and destabilization of PTEN protein involved in the cervical tumorigenesis. The STAT3 regulates PI3K/AKT signaling pathways and is involved in poor prognosis of cervical cancer. Moreover, various oncogenic signaling molecules and micro RNAs (miRNAs), small non-coding RNAs that modulate the expression of oncogenic and tumor-suppressive genes, which are play an important role in the development of cervical carcinogenesis. Thus targeting these oncogenic signaling pathways and miRNAs could be a novel approach for the treatment of cervical cancer (Page *et al.*, 2000; Wei *et al.*, 2001; Chen *et al.*, 2007; Wang *et al.*, 2008; Hou *et al.*, 2014; Prasad *et al.*, 2015; Lee *et al.*, 2015).

Arundhati Das *et al.*, (2018) have studied and the undertaken the investigation to ascertain the presence of anticancer Phyto-constituents in the Indian *Combretum* species and its further utilization in the treatment of tumor. The leaf extracts of *Combretum* species exhibited a higher quantity and anticancer activity than bark samples. The study further concludes as the methanolic leaf extract of *C. albidum* exhibited the highest percentage of chromosomal aberration such as the sticky bridge in metaphase, which demonstrated that the strongest cytotoxic effect in the root meristem cells.

The phytochemical study was conducted by Jamal *et al.* (2008), on the leaves of *Phyllanthus reticulatus* obtained from the riverside in Taman Negara Kuala Koh, Kelantan to separate and identify the chemical components by using different chromatographic techniques and the structures of compounds were elucidated by spectroscopic methods including nuclear magnetic resonance as well as mass spectrometry. The results indicate that three compounds were isolated and identified as lupeol acetate, stigmasterol and lupeol. Florence and Jeeva (2015) have studied the phytoconstituents present in *Gmelina asiatica* leaf through FTIR and GC-MS spectroscopy and isolated the bioconstituents. Tugba Artun *et al.* (2016) evaluated the *in vitro* anticancer and cytotoxic effect of methanolic extracts of 14 medicinal plants from different districts of Turkey, among these 8 plant species are endemic. The extracts were tested against the human HeLa cervical cancer cell line and to compare to the normal African green monkey kidney.

Sikander *et al.* (2016) investigated for the first time, *in vitro* and *in vivo* anti-cancer effects of a novel analogue of cucurbitacin D against cervical cancer and concluded the following aspects. Cucurbitacin D inhibited viability and growth of cervical cancer cells CaSki and SiHa with IC_{50} of 400 nM and 250 nM. Induction of apoptosis was observed in

Cucurbitacin D treated cervical cancer cells as measured by enhanced Annexin V staining and cleavage in PARP protein. Cucurbitacin D arrested the cell cycle in the G1/S phase, inhibited constitutive expression of E6, Cyclin D1, CDK4, pRb, and Rb and induced the protein levels of p21 and p27. In addition, they inhibited phosphorylation of STAT3 at Ser727 and Tyr705 residues as well as its downstream target genes c-Myc, and MMP9. Cucurbitacin D enhanced the expression of tumor suppressor microRNAs (miR-145, miRNA-143, and miRNA34a) in cervical cancer cells. Cucurbitacin D treatment (1 mg/kg body weight) effectively inhibited the growth of cervical cancer cells derived orthotopic xenograft tumors in athymic nude mice. These results demonstrate the potential therapeutic efficacy of Cucurbitacin D against cervical cancer.

The study conducted by Maqsood *et al.* (2018), on the salt range biodiversity of Pakistan and observed it has the rich floral diversity with the plant species belongs to Solanaceae family. Further, they have isolated myricetin, gallic acid, p-hydroxybenzoic acid and quercetin in leaf extract, leaf stalk extract and seed extract, respectively. From the *in vitro* study, it was observed as cytotoxic activity against human (HeLa, MCF-7, RD) and rat (RG2 and INS-1) cancer cell lines. Geetha and Vasuki (2019), investigated on the medicinally important plant species *Cissus quadrangularis* Linn. and the results revealed that methanolic extract of *C. quadrangularis* was more significant against cervical cancer when compared to ethanolic extract.

With the above scientific literature and background study, the present investigation was planned and taken up to study the ethnobotanical survey of Thiruvadisoolam village of Kanchipuram District, Tamil Nadu. Further, the physiochemical and pharmacological activities of selected medicinal plants from this area based on the ethnobotanical information also was evaluated. The present study, hope to provide necessary information on the exploration of medicinal plants for human welfare.

MATERIALS AND METHODS

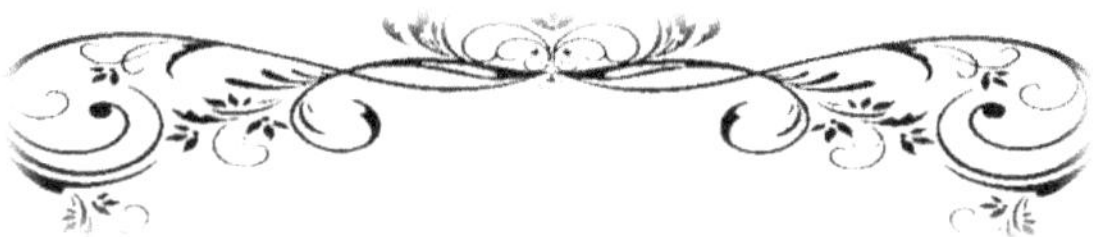

CHAPTER- III

MATERIALS AND METHODS

3.1 GLASSWARE AND CHEMICALS

All the glassware used throughout the experiments in the present study are belongs to Borosil Corning brand. They were soaked in chromic acid cleaning solution, then washed with detergent and rinsed in tap water, followed by distilled water. Analytical grade chemicals manufactured by Hi-Media, S.D. Fine Chemicals, Merck, Qualigens and Sigma Chemicals (U.S.A) were used for the various experiments carried out in the present study.

3.2 CLEANING OF GLASSWARE

All the glassware were immersed in a cleaning solution for few hours. Then, the glassware was washed thoroughly with tap water, followed by a detergent solution and finally rinsed with distilled water. The cleaned glassware were dried in a hot air oven and stored for further usage.

Cleaning solution (Mahadevan and Sridhar, 1996)

Potassium dichromate	-	60 g
Conc. H_2SO_4	-	60 ml
Distilled water	-	1000 ml

Potassium dichromate was dissolved in warm water, cooled and sulphuric acid was added slowly to make up to 1000 ml. It was mixed thoroughly and used for cleaning the glassware.

3.3 STUDY AREA DESCRIPTION

The study area selected for the present study is Thiruvadisoolam village, which is situated in Chengalpattu Thasil of Kanchipuram district, Tamil Nadu, which falls in south India (**Figure 2**).

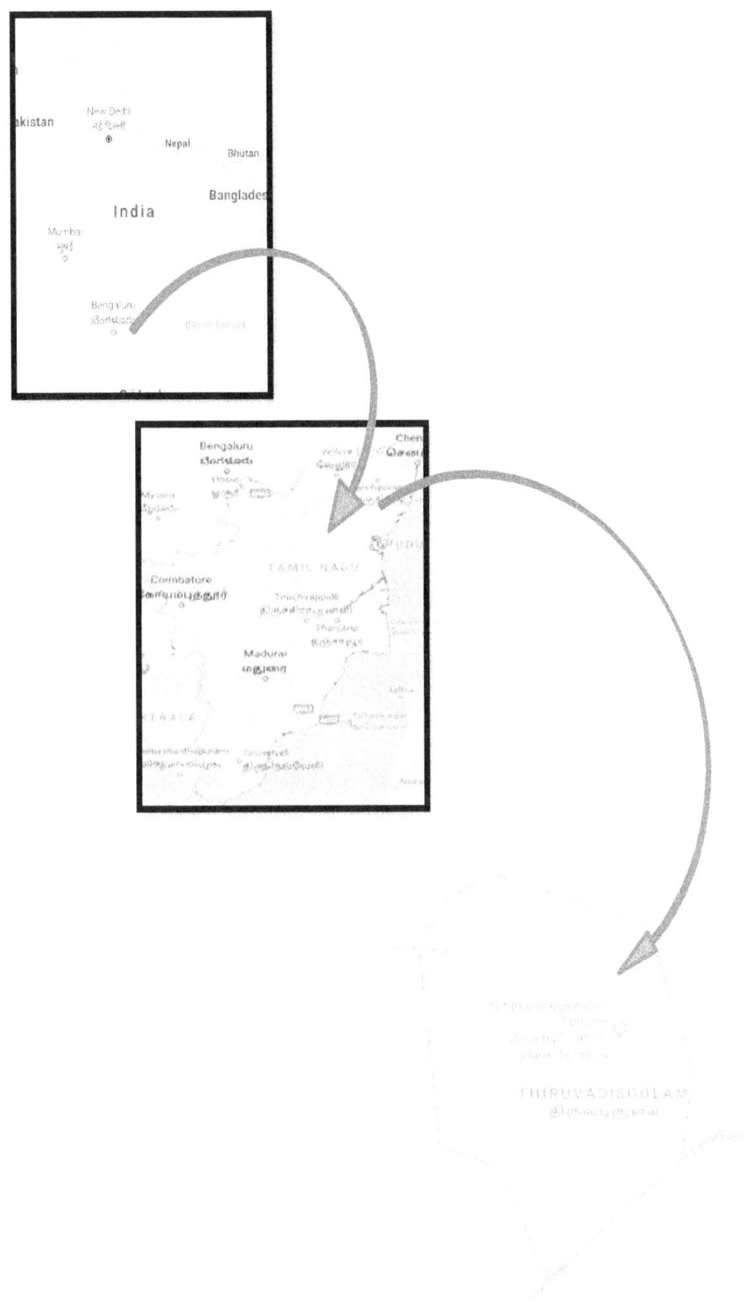

Figure 2. Map showing study area

35

The geographical coordinates of Thiruvadisoolam are latitude: 13.0938.995 and longitude: 80.292356. The geographical area of the village is 657.06 hectares. Thiruvadisoolam has nearly 1,500 people and the sex ratio is more are less equal in the percentage of the population. There are 300 houses in the village which the nearest town is Chengalpattu (10km away). The literacy rate of population in the village is 80%.

About 26% of the total geographical area is occupied by forest vegetation and more than 60% is utilized for agricultural and other purposes. A very small number of Tribal families reside in the village depend on forests for their needs like food, fodder, medicines, fire woods and timbers. They have a high assortment of indigenous traditional knowledge and medical practices in the conventional curative process.

3.4 METHODOLOGY FOR ETHNOBOTANICAL SURVEY

An ethnobotanical survey was conducted in Thiruvadisoolam village of Kanchipuram district to prepare a database on the medicinal plants used by the local peoples and tribes. The information about the medicinal uses of the plants to treat various diseases was documented from the herbal healers who were interested to disclose the information. Three basic approaches were adopted for the study.

A dialogue-based approach with a simple questionnaire was followed; in which questions are related to the usage of plants for various purposes (*i.e.*, medicine, food, fuel, fodder, etc.) was documented based on the informant during the visits to the forests for the collection of plant species and their identifications. An interactive dialogue approach was followed through meetings and discussions held with various stakeholders such as traditional herbal healers, school teachers, social workers, and the general public, to record the various uses of plants, methods and seasons of collection, and their conservation approaches and the providence of traditional knowledge systems, etc. The folklore knowledge about the uses of medicinal plants was also collected.

A preliminary field survey was conducted in the month of October 2014 to record the tribals and herbalists using plants as medicine for curative processes. Afterward, a list of local healers belonging to various segments was prepared for the information collected about medicinal plants used by them to cure various diseases. In the first phase of the meeting, all the herbalists were contacted and discussed on the program. In the same way, the second phase, those herbalists who ready to disclose their traditional knowledge were repeatedly interviewed between November-2014 and January-2016 to record the information in prepared formats (**Table 1**). The selected herbal healers were interviewed about the plants they used for medicinal purposes, the disease for which they use the plants, the parts which they use and the mode of application. Methods used to document the traditional knowledge included interviews, interactions, and inventory methods. Informants were chosen in the age of 21 to 60 years and there is no restriction for literacy status in the study area.Semi-structured interviews were conducted with the help of a questionnaire (Annexure I) provided to the healers and filled through face-to-face interviews with the help of local peoples. Each informant was interviewed individually so that they could provide independent information. The aim of the study was briefed before conducting the interviews.

The data such as plant parts used, preparation methods, the form of usage (fresh/dried), mode of application, as well as identification, collection and utilization were collected. Respondents were asked to state the degree of scarcity of the species and if there were any management and conservation activities in the particular area. In addition, observation and in-depth interviews with key informants, such as elder traditional healers, formed part of the field research. Regular field trips were made to the selected study area.

3.5 COLLECTION AND AUTHENTICATION OF PLANTS

Plant species of the study area were collected as per the standard procedure for respective plants and herbarium was prepared. The nomenclature of the plants collected was determined with the help of previously published works of literature, The Flora of Presidency of Madras (Gamble, 1935) and The Flora of Tamil Nadu Carnatic (Matthew, 1983). The collected plants were identified and authenticated by Prof. P. Jayaraman, Director, Institute of Herbal Botany, Plant Anatomy and Research Institute (PARC), West Tambaram, Chennai, Tamil Nadu, India. **Figure 3.** Shows the collection of plant species in Thiruvadisoolam forest with village people.

TABLE 1: LENGTH OF DATA COLLECTION

	Oct-14	Nov-14	Dec-14	Jan-15	Feb-15	Mar-15	Apr-15	May-15	Jun-15	Jul-15	Aug-15	Sep-15	Oct-15	Nov-15	Dec-15	Jan-16
Preliminary field survey	X															
Participant interviews		X	X	X	X											
Community observation						X	X	X	X							
Participant observation & transect walks		X	X	X	X	X	X	X	X							
Voucher specimen collection				X	X	X	X	X	X	X	X	X	X	X		
Identification and collection of plant samples														X	X	
Data analysis															X	X

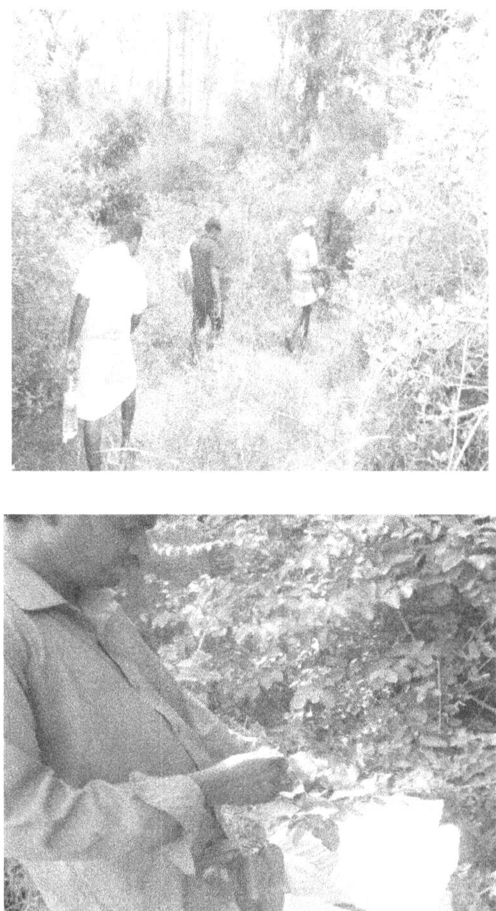

Figure 3. Collection of sample from Thiruvadisoolam

The systematic position, description of plant species and their pharmacological uses of selected 10 species of medicinally important plants were described in the following pages:

1. *Carissa spinarum* L.

Scientific classification

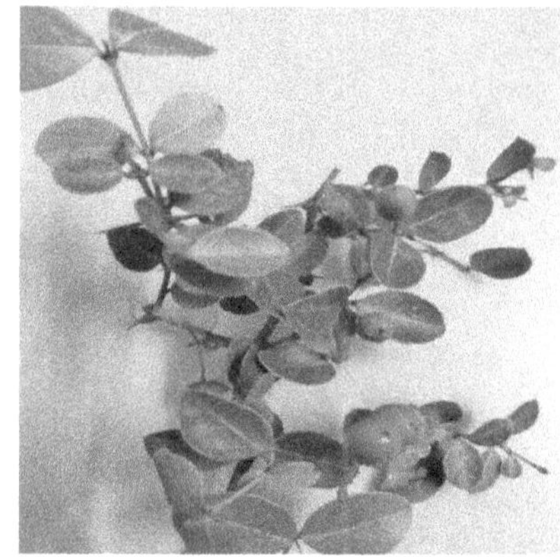

Figure 4. Habit of *Carissa spinarum* L.

Kingdom   : Plantae

Class   : Angiosperms

Sub Class   : Eudicots

Series   : Asterids

Order   : Gentianales

Family   : Apocynaceae

Genus   : *Carissa*

Species   : *spinarum*

Binomial name:*Carissa spinarum* L.

Description:

Medium shrub 1.5 to 2 m. The plant is ornamental and has dark green shiny leaves. The white flower is borne in bunches at the ends of branches. The stems are smooth and hard. Fruits start creamy white. They get a very pretty pink hue as they mature. They stay this way for over a month or two. They then mature to black. Fruit can be made into pickles, preserves and also candied. Plant growth can be quite haphazard. Regular and careful pruning is required to contain it. The spines make pruning difficult - but luckily this can be done every alternate year. Ladies in the Konkan area of Maharashtra traditionally wear a few fruits in their hair (**Figure 4**).

Pharmacology

Carissa spinarum fruits ready for consumption. The fruit is a rich source of iron, so it is sometimes used in the treatment of anemia. It contains a fair amount of Vitamin C and therefore is an antiscorbutic. Mature fruit is harvested for pickles. It contains pectin and accordingly is a useful ingredient in jelly, jam, syrup, and chutney. Ripe fruits exude white latex when severed from the branch. The roots of the plant are heavily branched, making it valuable for stabilizing eroding slopes. It has medicinal value too, it is taken for urine-related problems.

2. *Carmona retusa* (Vahl) Masamune

Scientific classification

Kingdom   : Plantae

Class   : Magnoliopsida

Subclass   : Asteridae

Order   : Lamiales

Family   : Boraginaceae

Genus   : *Carmona*

Species   : *retusa*

Binomial name : *Carmona retusa* (Vahl) Masamune

Description

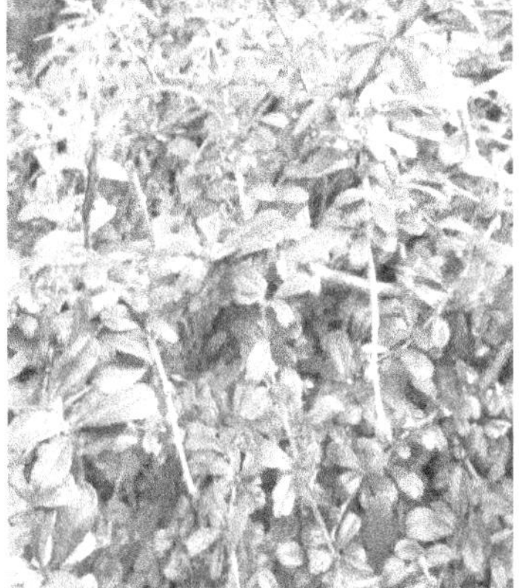

Figure 5. Habit of *Carmona retusa* (Vahl) Masamune

Evergreen shrub to a small tree. Leaves in clusters of 3-5, blade obovate or oblanceolate, 1.5-4 cm x .8-2.5 cm, base decurrent onto petiole, coarsely 3-5 toothed towards the apex, apex acute to obtuse or rounded, when young both surfaces with stiff white hairs, the upper surface becoming scabrid, petiole 1-5 mm long. Flowers 3-12 flowered scorpioid cymes, unbranched or branched once, sepals 4-5, lanceolate, 3-4 mm long; corolla white, rotate, 8-10 mm in diam., lobes 4-5, 3-4 mm long. Fruit globose, 4-5 mm in diameter, ripening brownish orange, pericarp thin, pyrene white, bony (**Figure 5**).

Pharmacology

The leaves are used medicinally in the Philippines to treat cough, colic, diarrhea and dysentery. The root is considered an antidote against plant-based poisoning and an alternative in cachexia and syphilis. Furthermore, it is traditionally used to stop the hemorrhaging resulting from the bite of the viper Echiscarinatus. The roots are reported to be ingested to clean the body after child birth. The plant has been shown to contain a range of medically active constituents. The leaves contain rosmarinic acid, flavonoid glycosides, and triterpenoids. Rosmarinic acid, a phenylacrylic acid derivative, is a known inhibitor of histamine release and a methanol extract of the leaves has shown strong antihistamine release properties.

3. *Combretum albidum* G. Don

Scientific classification

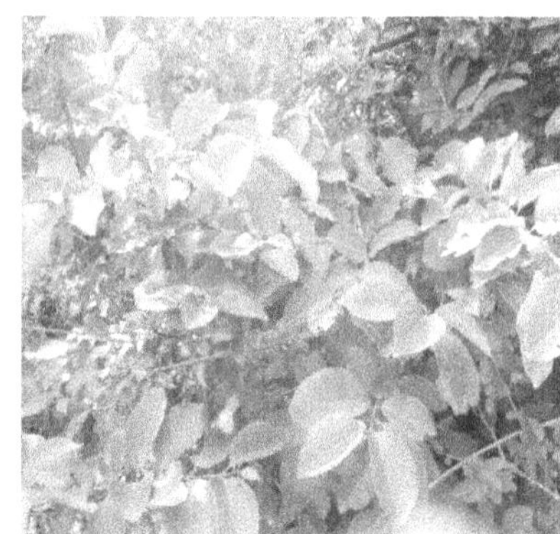

Kingdom   :Plantae

Class   : Angiosperms

Sub class   : Eudicots

Series   : Rosids

Order   : Myrtales

Family   : Combretaceae

Genus   : *Combretum.*

Species   : *albidum*

Binomial name: *Combretum albidum* G. Don

Figure 6. Habit of *Combretum albidum* G. Don

Description:

Leaves 7-10 x 5-6.5 cm, ovate, orbicular, apex acuminate; petiole to 1 cm. Spikes compound, axillary; flowers polygamy-dioceous, yellow; calyx tube constricted above, lobes 4, 1.5 mm, triangular; petals 1.5 mm, oblong-lanceolate, disc lining calyx pilose; stamens 8, in two rows, didymous, filaments 3 mm; ovary 3 mm, 1-loculed, style 3 mm, subulate. Fruit is 2 x 2 cm, 4-winged, wings chartaceous, red. The regional names are Tamil - Veragai, English - Buffalo calf plant, Malayalam – Manjakody, Marathi - PewarWel, Piluki, Pilokha, Others MenthaiKodi, UlavaiMaram, Piluki, Dhavshira, Okha, Oval-leaved Wheel Creeper, Manjakody, Odaikodi, OdaiKodi, Verragay, Vennangukodi, Telugu - Geddepeyyeru, ShirtalBoddi, Yada-tige, Putangi (**Figure 6**).

Pharmacology

C. albidum afforded five triterpenoids namely ursolic acid, oleanolic acid, betulinic acid, arjunolic acid, and betulin. The heartwood of the plant also yields beta-sitosterol, gallic acid, and ellagic acid as other constituents. The compounds oleanolic acid, betulinic acid, arjunolic acid, betulin, and ellagic acid are major components present in the plant.

4. *Cassia auriculata* L.

Scientific classification

Kingdom : Plantae

Class : Angiosperms

Sub Class : Eudicots

Series : Rosids

Order : Fabales

Family : Fabaceae

Genus : *Cassia*

Species : *auriculata*

Binomial name: *Cassia auriculata* (L.)

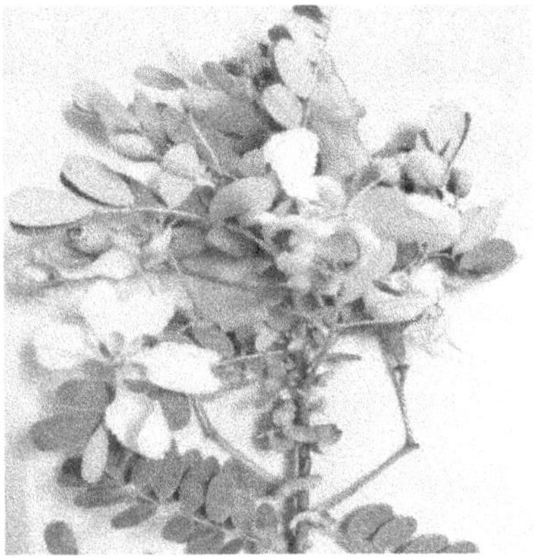

Description

Figure 7. Habit of *Cassia auriculata* L.

A shrub occurring in Madhya Pradesh, West Bengal, Tamil Nadu and Rajasthan. Mostly present in dry places, stony hills and black soil. The leaves are Mucronate, alternate leaf arrangement, leaf bases are Cuneate, leaf margins are entire, oblanged, parpinate. Leaflets with glands on rachis or petiole and foliaceous stipules. Flowrers are beautiful bright large yellow flowers with axillary or terminal corymbose racemes and flowering throughout the year. The fruits are long pod, flat, stipitate, turgid and apices obtuse, brown when adult. Fruiting during throughout the year and the seeds are presented above 6 and ovoid in brown (**Figure 7**).

Pharmacology

The plant is used in Ayurveda in the treatment of diabetes. The flower and leaf extract of *C. auriculata* is shown as antihyperglycemic in streptozotocin-induced experimental diabetes. Methanolic extracts of *C. auriculata* flowers have been demonstrated to inhibit α-glucosidase *in vivo* as well as *in vitro*. Its aqueous extract is reported to prevent lipid peroxidation in the brain of diabetic rats. Hyponid, a formulation containing *C. auriculata* has been shown as antihyperglycemic and antioxidant. Flavonoids, β-sitosterol-β-d-glucoside, polysaccharides, anthracene, dimericprocyanidins and myristyl alcohol, were other components present in the plant parts.

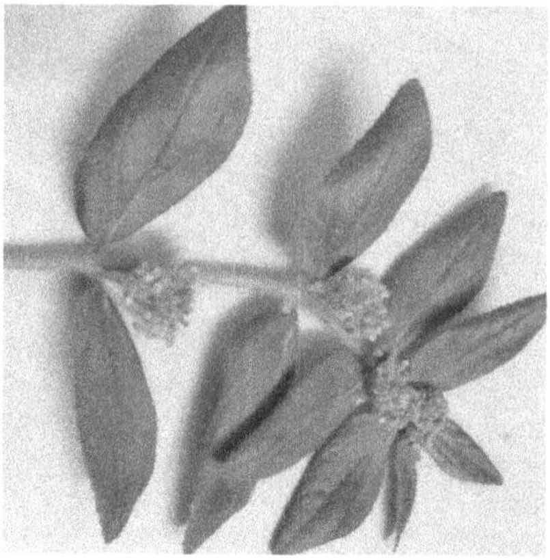

5. *Euphorbia hirta* L.

Scientific classification

Kingdom : Plantae

Class : Angiosperms

Sub Class : Eudicots

Series : Rosids

Order : Malpighiales

Family : Euphorbiaceae

Genus : *Euphorbia*

Species : *hirta*

Binomial name: *Euphorbia hirta* L.

Description

Figure 8. Habit of *Euphorbia hirta* L.

This erect or prostrate annual herb can get up to 60 cm long with a solid, hairy stem that produced abundant white latex. stipules present, leaves are simple, elliptical, hairy (on both upper and lower surfaces but particularly on the veins on the lower leaf surface), with a finely dentate margin. Leaves occur in opposite pairs on the stem. The flowers are unisexual and found in axillary cymes at each leaf node. They lack petals and are generally on a stalk. The fruit is a capsule with three valves and produces tiny, oblong, four-sided red seeds. It has a white or brown taproot. *E. hirta* is distributed throughout the hotter parts of India and Australia, often found in waste places along the roadsides (**Figure 8**).

Pharmacology

An alcoholic extract of *E. hirta* leaves is highly effective against gram-positive bacteria and moderately effective against gram-negative bacteria. The diuretic effects of leaf extracts were assessed using Acetazolamide (Diamox) and Furosemide (Lasix) as standard diuretic drugs. It produced a time-dependent increase in urine output and electrolyte excretion was also significantly affected by the plant extracts. This study suggests that the active components in the water extract of *E. hirta* leaf had a similar diuretic spectrum to that of acetazolamide.

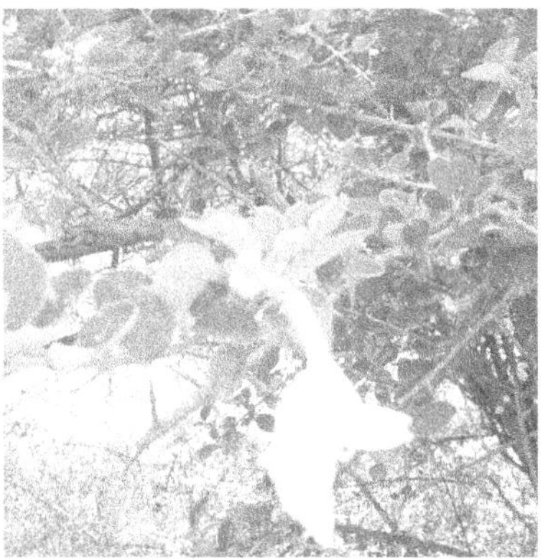

6. *Gmelina asiatica* L.

Scientific classification

Kingdom   : Plantae

Class   : Magnoliopsida

Subclass   : Asteridae

Order   : Lamiales

Family   : Verbenaceae

Genus   : *Gmelina*

Species   : *asiatica*

Binomial name: *Gmelina asiatica* L.

Figure 9. Habit of *Gmelina asiatica* L.

Description

Shrubs, climbing, 1–3 m tall, usually with spines and minute yellowish-brown hairs on young shoots. Petiole 0.5–4.5 cm; leaf blade ovate to subovate, papery, abaxially dark brown villous and glandular, adaxially glabrescent, base cuneate, margin entire lobed, apex acuminate, veins 3 or 4 pairs. Inflorescences terminal, usually pendulous, primary floral branches very short, 1–5-flowered; bracts leaflike, small to large. Flowers pendulous. Calyx 3–6 × 2.5–4 mm, outside densely dark brown pubescent and with 2 to several disc-shaped glands, inside glabrous. Corolla yellow, 2–5 cm, 2-lipped and 4-lobed, lower lip 3-lobed, upper lip entire, outside with scattered appressed hairs, inside with dense glandular hairs.

Filaments with dense glandular hairs. Ovary 4-locular, glabrous. Style slender, hardly exerted, apically curved; stigma unequally 2-cleft. Drupes yellow, ovoid to obovoid, glabrous (**Figure 9**).

Pharmacology

Roots, bark, fruit, leaves, and young shoots are traditionally used as various medicinal properties like anti-inflammatory, cancer preventive, hepatoprotective, nematicide, insectifuge, antihistaminic, antieczemicantieczemic, antiacne, 5-alpha reductase inhibitor, and hypocholesterolemic agent. It was reported that leaves and aerial parts are used in the treatment of jaundice, body heat and other hepatic diseases as reported by tribal people.

7. *Kirganelia reticulate* (Poir) Baill

Scientific classification

Kingdom   : Plantae

Class   : Angiosperms

Sub Class   : Eudicots

Series   : Rosids

Order   : Malpighiales

Family   : Phyllanthaceae

Genus   : *Kirganelia*

Species   : *reticulata*

Binomial name: *Kirganelia reticulata* (Poir) Baill

Description   **Figure 10. Habit of *Kirganelia reticulata* (Poir) Baill**

A large branched and scandent shrub with branches smooth or tuberculate and somewhat angled. Leaves have an alternate arrangement, lanceolate, simple and variable in size. The apex of the leaves is acute, ventral side is dark green in color while the dorsal side is light-green. It is having a bitter taste and pungent odor. Leaves are 2.5-5 cm long and 0.7-1.5 cm broad, oblong and elliptic in shape. The margins of the leaves are emarginated to undulate. Flowers are axillary on slender branches. Fruits are coriaceous or fleshy and 8-16 seeded. Seeds are irregularly trigonous (**Figure 10**).

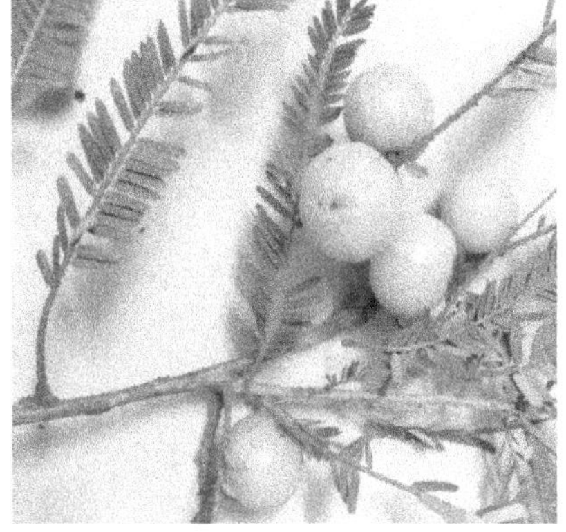

Regional name

Sanskrit - Pulika, Krishna-kamboji, Bengali – Panjulil, Gujarati – Datwan, Hindi – Panjuli, Kannada - Pulaveri, Anamsule, Malayalam - Niruri, Nireli, Marathi – Pavana, Oriya – Jandaki, Tamil - Abaranji, Karunelli, Kattukilanelli, Telugu - allapurugudu

Pharmacology

Three compounds such as stigmasterol, lupeol and lupeol acetate were reported to have isolated and identified by a phytochemical produces on the leaves of *K. reticulata*.

8. *Phyllanthus emblica* L.

Scientific classification

Kingdom   : Plantae

Class   : Angiosperms

Sub Class   : Eudicots

Series   : Rosids

Order   : Malpighiales

Family   : Phyllanthaceae

Genus   : *Phyllanthus*

Species   : *emblica*

Binomial name: *Phyllanthus emblica* L.

Figure 11. Habit of *Phyllanthus emblica* L.

Description

The tree is small to medium in size, reaching 1–8 m (3ft 3 in–26 ft 3 in) in height. The branchlets aren't glabrous or finely pubescent, 10–20 cm (3.9–7.9 in) long, usually deciduous; the leaves are simple, subsessile and closely set along branchlets, light green, resembling pinnate leaves. The flowers are greenish-yellow. The fruit is nearly spherical, light greenish-yellow, quite smooth and hard on appearance, with six vertical stripes or furrows. Ripening in autumn, the berries are 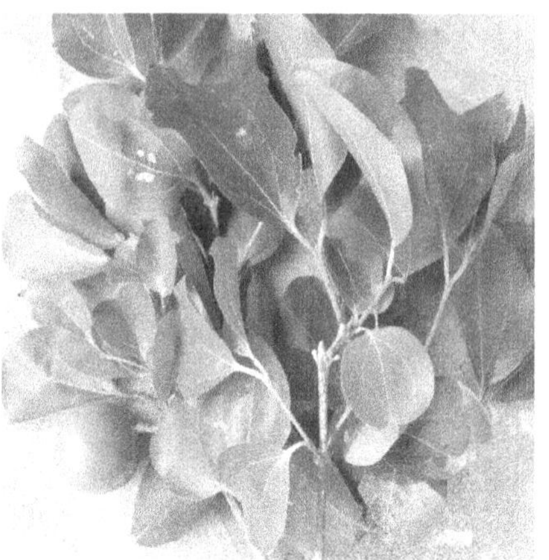 harvested by hand after climbing to upper branches bearing the fruits. The taste of Indian gooseberry is sour, bitter and astringent, and it is quite fibrous. In India, it is common to eat gooseberries steeped in saltwater and red chili powder to make the sour fruits palatable **(Figure 11)**.

Pharmacology

Although these fruits are reputed to contain high amounts of ascorbic acid (vitamin C), up to 445 mg per 100 g, the specific contents are disputed, and the overall antioxidant strength of amla may derive instead from its high density of ellagi tannins such as emblicanin A (37%), emblicanin B (33%), punigluconin (12%) and pedunculagin (14%).It also contains punicafolin and phyllanemblinin A, phyllanemblin other polyphenols: flavonoids, kaempferol, ellagic acid and gallic acid.

9. *Strychnos nux-vomica* L.

Scientific classification

Kingdom   : Plantae

Class   : Angiosperms

Sub Class   : Eudicots

Series   : Asterids

Order   : Gentianales

Family   : Loganiaceae

Genus   : *Strychnos*

Species   : *nux-vomica*

Binomial name: *Strychnos nux-vomica* L.

Description

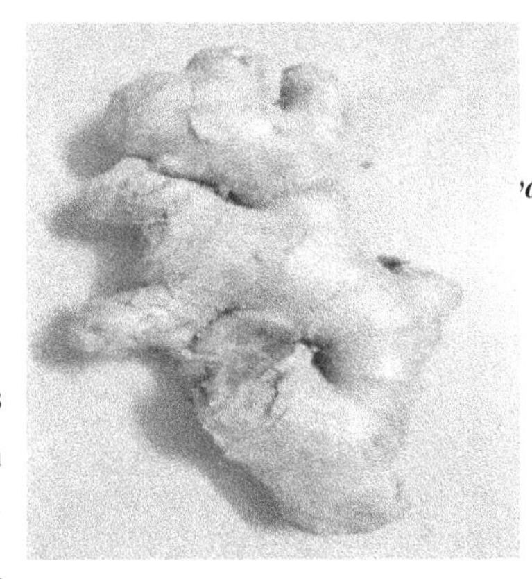

The *S. nux-vomica* L. also known as strychnine tree, nux vomica, poison nut, semen strychnos, and quaker buttons, is a deciduous tree native to India, and Southeast Asia. It is a medium-sized tree in the family Loganiaceae that grows in open habitats. Its leaves are ovate and 2–3.5 inches (5.1–8.9 cm) in size. It is a major source of the highly poisonous, intensely bitter alkaloids strychnine and brucine, derived from the seeds inside the tree's round, green to orange fruit. The seeds contain approximately 1.5% strychnine, and the dried blossoms contain 1.0%. However, the tree's bark also contains brucine and other poisonous compounds **(Figure 12)**.

Pharmacology

Bark of *S. nux-vomica* is promoted within herbal medicine as being a treatment for cancer and heart disease. Since the seeds contain strychnine poison, conventional doctors do not recommend it as a medicine. It is on the Commission E-list of unapproved herbs because it is not recommended for use and has not been proven to be safe or effective. In the Indian (Ayush) system of medicine.

10. *Zingiber officinale* Roscoe

Scientific classification

Kingdom   : Plantae

Class   : Angiosperms

Sub Class   : Monocots

Series   : Commelinids

Order   : Zingiberales

Family   : Zingiberaceae

Genus   : *Zingiber*

Species   : *officinale*

Binomial name: *Zingiber officinale* Roscoe

Figure 13. Habit of *Zingiber officinale* Roscoe

Description:

It is a herbaceous perennial which grows annual stems about a meter tall bearing narrow green leaves and yellow flowers. Ginger is in the family Zingiberaceae, to which also belong turmeric (Curcuma longa), cardamom (Elettariacardamomum), and galangal. Ginger originated in the lush tropical jungles in Southern Asia. Although ginger no longer grows wild, it is thought to have originated on the Indian subcontinent. The larger the number of genetic variations, the longer the plant has grown in that region. Ginger was exported to Europe via India in the first century AD as a result of the lucrative spice trade and was used extensively by the Romans (**Figure 13**).

Pharmacology

The characteristic odor and flavor of ginger is caused by a mixture of zingerone, shogaols, gingerols and volatile oils. The pungent taste of ginger is due to nonvolatile phenylpropanoid-derived compounds, particularly gingerols and shogaols, which form from gingerols when ginger is dried or cooked. Zingerone is also produced from gingerols, this compound is less pungent and has a spicy-sweet aroma.

3.6 PREPARATION AND STORAGE OF PLANT MATERIAL

All the plant material collected were washed with the water, followed by 75% ethanol to prevent deterioration and dried during under shade until complete removal of water is achieved. Then the dried plant materials were powdered by using laboratory pulverizer and sieved through mesh. Finally the powdered material was stored in an airtight container for further use.

3.7 PREPARATION OF PLANT CRUDE EXTRACTS

The powdered plant material 10 g was soaked in 100 ml of methanol and kept at room temperature for 72 hours in a shaker. Then the mixture is filtered through whatmann No.1 filter paper and the filtrate was collected. The above procedure was repeated thrice and the filtrate were collected and condensed by using a rotary evaporator in a vacuum. The concentrated crude extract was collected and stored in a glass vial after properly labelled (**Figure 14**).

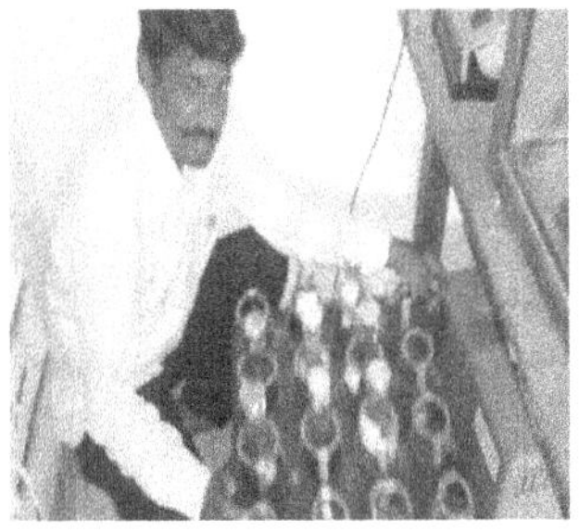

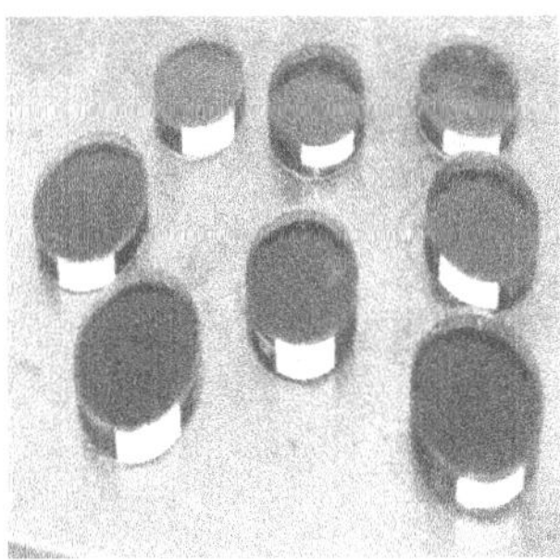

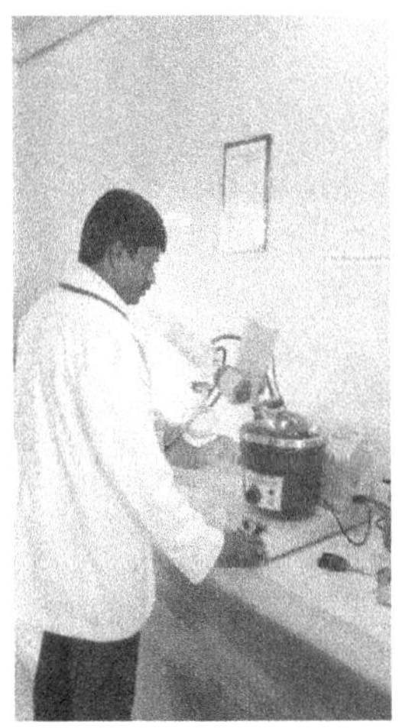

Figure 14: Crude extract preparation (a) extraction of metabolites under shaking condition, (b) Condensing of obtained extracts using vacuum evaporator and (c) Air drying of condensed extracts

3.8 QUALITATIVE PHYTOCHEMICAL ANALYSIS

Exactly 10% of the concentrated crude methanol extract of different plant parts such as leaf and rhizome was used for qualitative screening of phytochemical compounds *viz.*, alkaloids, anthraquinones, coumarins, flavonoids, glycosides, phenols, saponins, steroids, tannins, and terpenoids in accordance with the standard methods (Trease and Evans, 1989; Harborne, 1998).

3.8.1. Alkaloids (Mayer's test)

Exactly 0.5 g of the crude methanol extract was stirred with a few milliliters of dilute hydrochloric acid and filtered. To a few milliliters of filtrate, one or two drops of Mayer's reagent were added along the sides of the test tube. A white creamy precipitate demonstrated the test as positive.

3.8.2. Reducing sugars Fehling's test.

The extract (100mg) was dissolved in 5ml of water and filtered. About 1ml of the filtrate was boiled on a water bath with 1ml each of Fehling's solution I and II. A red precipitate indicates the presence of reducing sugars.

3.8.3. Steroids (Salkwoski's test)

Exactly 0.5 g of the extract was dissolved in 2 ml of chloroform. Sulfuric acid was then carefully added to form a lower layer. A reddish-brown color at the interface indicated the presence of steroids.

3.8.4. Terpenoids (Hishorn's test)

The crude methanol extract 0.5 g was dissolved in 2 ml of chloroform. The mixture was heated for 10 min, after the addition of 2 ml trichloroacetic acid. The change of yellow color to red indicates the presence of triterpenoids.

3.8.5. Flavonoids (Ferric chloride test)

Exactly 0.5 g of the crude methanol extract was boiled with distilled water and then filtered. To 2 ml of the filtrate, a few drops of 10% ferric chloride solution were then added. The formation of green-blue or violet coloration indicated the presence of flavonoids.

3.8.6. Phenols (Lead acetate test)

About 0.5 g of the crude methanolic extract was treated with lead acetate solution. The formation of precipitate indicated the presence of phenols.

3.8.7. Glycosides (Salkwoski's test)

About 0.5 g of the crude methanolic extract was dissolved in 2 ml of chloroform. Sulfuric acid was then carefully added to form a lower layer. A reddish-brown color at the interface demonstrated the presence of glycosides.

3.8.8. Saponin (Frothing test)

To 1 g of the crude methanolic extract and 3 ml of distilled water was mixed and shaken vigorously for 5 minutes. Frothing which persisted on warming was taken as a piece of evidence for the presence of saponins.

3.8.9. Tannins

Exactly 1.0 g of leaf extract was dissolved in 10 ml of distilled water and filtered using Whatman No. 1 filter paper. A blue coloration resulting followed by the addition of ferric chloride reagent to the filtrate indicated the presence of tannins in the extract.

3.8.10. Proteins (Biuret test)

An aliquot of 2 ml of filtrate was treated with one drop of 2% copper sulphate solution. To this, 1 ml of ethanol (95%) was added, followed by an excess of potassium hydroxide pellets. The pink colour in the ethanolic layer indicated the presence of proteins.

3.9 QUANTITATIVE PHYTOCHEMICAL ANALYSIS

3.9.1 DETERMINATION OF TOTAL PHENOLIC CONTENT (Mavi *et al.*, 2004)

The total content of the phenolic compounds in the methanol extract of the above 10 plants was determined by Folin-Ciocalteu's method (Mavi *et al.*, 2004) gallic acid as a standard. Folin-Ciocalteu's phenol reagent 250 µL was mixed with 50 µL of the sample and 500 µL of 20% water solution of Na_2CO_3 was added to the mixture. Mixtures were vortexed and completed with water to 5 ml. As a control, reagent without adding extract was used. After incubation of the samples at room temperature for 30 min, their absorbance was measured at 765 nm. The calibration curve created by using freshly prepared gallic acid solutions was used as a base in calculations of total phenolic compound contents in the extracts.

3.9.2 DETERMINATION OF TOTAL FLAVONOID CONTENT (Ordonez *et al.*, 2006)

The total flavonoid content of methanol extract of 10 plant parts was determined by using aluminium chloride ($AlCl_3$) method (Ordonez *et al.*, 2006) and quercetin were used as a standard. The plant methanol extract (0.1 ml) was added to 0.3 ml distilled water followed by 5% $NaNO_2$ (0.03 ml). After 5 min at 25°C, $AlCl_3$ (0.03 ml, 10%) was added. After a further 5 min, the reaction mixture was treated with 0.2 ml of 1 mM NaOH. Finally, the reaction mixture was diluted to 1 ml with water and the absorbance was measured at 510 nm. The results were expressed as mg quercetin (QE)/g in comparison.

3.10 ANTIMICROBIAL STUDIES (Chew *et al.*, 2011)

Many plants have provided essential clues for being used as potentially, fungicidal and antibacterial compounds. In accordance with this information, Methanolic plant extracts of *Zingiber officinale, Carrissa spinarium, Euphorbia hirta, Strychnosnux-vomica, Phyllanthus embilica, Gmelina asiatica, Cassia auriculata, Carmona retusa, Kirganelia reticulata* and *Combretum albidum* were subjected to test antibacterial nature against different bacterial strains.

3.10.1 MICROBIAL STRAINS

The standard strains of two Gram-Positive Bacteria namely *Bacillus subtilis* (MTCC - 441), *Micrococcus luteus* (MTCC - 1538) and two gram-negative bacterial strains namely *Proteus mirabilis* (MTCC- 426), *Salmonella typhii* (MTCC 25923) were obtained from the Department of Medical Microbiology, Institute of Basic Medical Sciences, Taramani Campus, University of Madras, Chennai, Tamil Nadu for the present study. All the aforesaid test bacterial species were maintained on the Nutrient Agar (NA) medium for further experiments.

3.10.2 MEDIA COMPOSITION NUTRIENT AGAR (NA)

Ingredients	Quantity
Sodium chloride	5.0 g
Peptone	5.0 g
Yeast extract	3.0 g
Agar	20.0 g
Double distilled water	1000 ml
pH	7.4±0.2

3.10.3 INHIBITION ASSAY (DISC-DIFFUSION METHOD)

Nutrient Agar medium was prepared as per the above composition, poured into a conical flask and sterilized by autoclaving at 121°C and 15lb pressure for 20 min. The culture medium was then poured into Petri plates (10 cm diameter) at room temperature and let to stand for around 20 min for solidification. Whatman No.1 Filter paper discs of 4 mm diameter were made and sterilized. The discs were taken and impregnated with respective methanolic plant extracts. Sample loaded discs were dried and placed over agar plates (equidistance from each other and the circumference of the plate) with the test organisms and incubated at desired conditions of 37 °C in an incubator. Then the inoculated plates were allowed in incubator for 24 hrs to 48 hrs period. Clear zones of growth inhibition around the discs on the agar medium stand for antibacterial nature. Triplicates of the extracts were run for standardizing the result. The resulting zone of inhibition was measured in mm using a scale. The zones of growth inhibitions around the discs were measured and the area of inhibition was calculated. Simultaneously, the activity of standard antibiotic Streptomycin was also tested against the microorganisms under study in similar conditions, so as to compare the degree of inhibition. Discs fed with corresponding solvents served as controls. The Zone of Inhibition is the mean of the values obtained (Chew *et al.*, 2011).

3.11 DETERMINATION OF ANTIOXIDANT ACTIVITY

3.11.1 DPPH RADICAL SCAVENGING ASSAY (Raaman, 2006)

The DPPH free radical scavenging activity of methanol extract of the ten different plant species was carried out according to the method of Raaman, (2006). One ml of Plant methanol extract of various concentrations (10, 20, 40, 80, 160, 320 µg/ml) were mixed with 1 ml of 0.1 mM DPPH solution in acetone. The reaction mixture was kept in dark at room temperature for 30 min. Absorbance was read at 517 nm in a spectrophotometer. Ascorbic acid was used as the standard for reference. The percentage of radical scavenging activity was calculated as follows.

$$\% \text{ of DPPH inhibition} = \frac{\text{control - sample}}{\text{control}} \times 100$$

3.11.2 PHOSPHOMOLYBDENUM REDUCTION ASSAY (Prieto *et al.*, 1999).

The Phospho-molybdenum reduction assays were determined for the above ten plant species as described by Prieto *et al.* (1999). One ml of different concentration of the extract (10- 320 µg/ml) was taken and 1.0 ml of the reagent (0.6 M sulphuric acid, 28 mM sodium phosphate and 4 mM ammonium molybdate) was added. The tubes were capped and incubated in a water bath at 95°c for 90 min. Ascorbic acid was used as a standard. The absorbance was measured at 695 nm against a blank after cooling at room temperature.

3.11.3 Fe^{3+} REDUCING POWER ASSAY (Oyaizu, 1986)

The reducing power of crude methanol extract of ten plants was determined by the method of Oyaizu, (1986). Various concentrations of the plant extracts (10, 20, 40, 80, 160, 320 µg/ml) in 1.0 ml of solvent were mixed with phosphate buffer (2.5 ml) and potassium ferricyanide (2.5 ml) and incubated at 50°C for 20 min. Trichloroacetic acid (2.5 ml) was added to the mixture, which was then centrifuged at 3000 rpm for 10 min whenever necessary. The upper layer of solution (2.5 ml) was mixed with distilled water (2.5 ml) and a freshly prepared ferric chloride solution (0.5 ml). The absorbance was measured at 700 nm. A blank was prepared without adding plant extract. Ascorbic acid with various concentrations was used as the standard reference. An increase in absorbance of the reaction mixture indicates an increase in reducing power of the plant methanolic crude compounds.

3.12 PHARMOCOGNOSTIC STUDIES

3.12.1 COLLECTION OF PLANT SPECIMENS

The plant species specimens for this study were collected from Thiruvadisoolam village of Kanchipuram district, South India based on the ethnobotanical survey. Care was taken to select healthy plants with normal plant organ. The required samples of different organs were cut and removed from the plant and fixed in FAA (5ml Farmalin+ 5ml Acetic acid + 90ml of 70% Ethyl alcohol). After 24 hrs of fixing, the specimens were dehydrated with a graded series of tertiary –Butyl alcohol as per the schedule is given by Sass (1940). Infiltration of the specimens was carried by the gradual addition of paraffin wax (melting point 58-60 °C) until the TBA solution attained super saturation. The specimens were cast into paraffin blocks.

3.12.2 PHYTOANATOMICAL STUDIES

The arrangement of cells and tissue systems of plants indicates their specialized nature and knowledge of their micro morphological features is a salient requirement of the scientific study of plant drugs to establish their identity.

3.12.3 SECTIONING

The paraffin-embedded specimens were sectioned with the help of Rotary Microtome. The thickness of the sections was 10-12 µm. Dewaxing of the sections was by the customary procedure (Johansen, 1940). The sections were stained with Toluidine blue as per the method published by O'Brien et al. (1964). Since Toluidine blue is a polychromatic stain, the staining results were remarkably good, and some cytochemical reactions were also obtained. The dye rendered pink color to the cellulose walls, blue to the lignified cells, dark green to suberin, violet to the mucilage, blue to the protein bodies, etc. Wherever necessary sections were also stained with safranin and Fast-green and Potassium Iodide (for Starch)

For studying the stomatal morphology, venation pattern and trichome distribution, paradermal sections (sections were taken parallel to the surface of the leaf) as well as clearing of the leaf with 5% sodium hydroxide or epidermal peeling by partial maceration employing Jeffrey's maceration fluid (Sass, 1940) were prepared. Glycerine mounted temporary preparations were made for macerated/cleared materials. Powdered materials of different parts were cleared with NaOH and mounted in glycerine medium after staining. Different cell component were studied and measured.

3.12.4 PHOTOMICROGRAPHS

Microscopic descriptions of tissues are supplemented with micrographs wherever necessary. Photographs of different magnifications were taken with the Nikon lab photo 2 microscopic Unit. For normal observations, the bright field was used. For the study of crystals, starch grains and lignified cells, polarized light was employed. Since these structures have birefringent property, under polarized light they appear bright against a dark background. Magnifications of the figures are indicated by the scale-bars. Descriptive terms of the anatomical features are as given in the standard Anatomy books (Esau, 1964).

3.12.5 PROXIMATE ANALYSIS

Proximate analysis concerning the assessment of ash and extractive values of a crude drug is a means for the evaluation of crude drugs, the establishment of genuineness, and ruling out all forms of tarnishing. While extractive values provide a process of an assay for drugs that are not readily estimated by other means, determination of ash values is useful for detecting low-grade products, exhausted drugs, and the presence of sandy and earthy matter. The following are the parameters studied.

3.12.5.1 ASH VALUE DETERMINATION

Incineration of vegetable drugs, all organic matters are oxidized and removed leaving inorganic ash. Total ash consisting mainly of chlorides, carbonates, phosphates, silicates and silica, is used to detect adherent earthy matter. Water-soluble ash detects the presence of material exhausted by water. Acid insoluble ash detects the presence of earthy matter in drugs with ash values varying within fairly wide limits, for example, drugs rich in calcium oxalate.

3.12.5.2 TOTAL ASH

The sample from 2g of crude drug powder accurately weighed was incinerated in a tared silica crucible at a temperature not exceeding 450°C by using muffle furnace, until free from carbon, cooled and weighed. The percentage of ash was calculated with reference to the air-dried drug.

3.12.5.3 WATER-SOLUBLE ASH

The ash was boiled for 5 min with 25 ml distilled water. The insoluble matter was collected on an ashless filter paper, washed with hot water and ignited for 15 min at a temperature not exceeding 450° C by using muffle furnance. The weight of the insoluble matter was subtracted from the weight of the ash. The difference in weight represents the water-soluble ash and the percentage of water-soluble ash with reference to the air-dried drug was calculated.

3.12.5.4 ACID-INSOLUBLE ASH

The ash was boiled with 25 ml of 2M HCl for 5 min. Insoluble matter was collected on an ashless filter paper, washed with hot water, ignited, cooled in a desiccator and weighed. The percentage of acid-insoluble ash was calculated with reference to the air-dried drug.

3.12.5.5 EXTRACTIVE VALUE DETERMINATION

Extractive tests are required as Pharmacopeia standards, for official drugs for which suitable assays are not available. The yield to solvents, provide a means of detecting and approximately determining the amount of an adulterant which yields matter to a solvent that has little or no action upon the drug itself. The amount of insoluble matter also will indicate the presence of an unreasonable amount of extraneous vegetable matter. Extractive values with water, methanol and dichloromethane solvents, may also serve as standardization

3.12.5.6 METHANOL-SOLUBLE EXTRACTIVE VALUE

Five grams of accurately weighed, air-dried, then coarsely powdered drug was completely extracted with the solvent and aqueous at room temperature. Methanol and water extracts represent total extracts. The extracts were filtered through Whatman filter paper no: 1 and distilled on a water bath in a rotary vacuum evaporator and dried in vacuum to constant weight.

3.12.5.7 MOISTURE CONTENT

Five gram of leaf powdered crude drug was accurately weighed in a tared dish and dried in an oven at 105°C for 1 hr. It was cooled in a desiccator and weighed. The Moisture content was calculated with reference to the amount of dried powder taken.

3.12.5.8 FLUORESCENCE ANALYSIS

The fluorescence analysis of the powdered plant drug material from the leaves of *C. albidum*in with various solvents and chemical reagents was performed under normal and Ultra Violet (UV) light. The fluorescent colour reflected by the drug was noticed.

3.13 ISOLATION AND PURIFICATION OF BIOACTIVE COMPOUNDS

3.13.1 THIN LAYER CHROMATOGRAPHY

Thin layer chromatography (TLC) is used to separate components from a mixture or crude sample material. The stationary phase consists of silica gel pre coated in aluminium sheet and the mobile phase was different solvent system. The crude extract and eluted fractions were spotted at the bottom of the TLC plate above 0.5 cm and kept for 5 min at room temperature to dry. The TLC plate was subjected to run with a particular solvent system in the developing chamber. The solvent system moves upward and crossing the sample by capillary action. The reaction was stopped at below 0.5 cm of the top of the TLC plate. The components were separated between the stationary and mobile phase and the R_f value of separated components were determined by using the following formula:

$$R_f \text{ value} = \frac{\text{Distance traveled by the component}}{\text{Distance traveled by the component}} \times 100$$

3.13.2 C

The activation of silica gel (100-200 mesh size) was kept at 110°C for 1 hr. The silica gel slurry was formed by using hexane and allowed to vigorous stirring to eliminate the air. The bottom of the glass column (40mm x 400mm) cotton was placed to keep away from exhausting of silica gel and the silica gel slurry was poured into a column with modest tapping for tight and uniform packing. The setup contains a small amount of hexane that remains above the silica gel to avoid air cracks. Then 30 g of *C. albidum* methanolic extract was dispensed into the column by using glass funnel. The settled extract was eluted with a mobile phase of hexane solvent (non-polar), ethyl acetate with a gradual increase of volume of a higher polar solvent. The flow rate of elution was 1 ml min^{-1} with gradient 100 ml of hexane: ethyl acetate (9:1 to 0:10) and ethyl acetate: methanol (9:1 to 0:10), finally the column was eluted with 100% methanol to washout the residues.

3.14 CHARACTERIZATION OF ISOLATED BIOACTIVE COMPOUND

3.14.1 GAS CHROMATOGRAPHY - MASS SPECTRUM (GC-MS) ANALYSIS

The Clarus 680 Gas Chromatography was used in the analysis employed a fused silica column, packed with Elite-5MS (5% biphenyl 95% dimethylpolysiloxane, 30 m × 0.25 mm ID × 250μm df) and the components were separated using Helium as carrier gas at a constant flow of 1 ml/min. The injector temperature was set at 260°C during the chromatographic run. The 1μL of extract sample injected into the instrument with the oven temperature was as follows: 60 °C (2 min); followed by 300 °C at the rate of 10 °C min−1; and 300 °C, where it was held for 6 min. The mass detector conditions were: transfer line temperature 240 °C; ion source temperature 240 °C; and ionization mode electron impact at 70 eV, scan time 0.2 sec and scan interval of 0.1 sec. The fragments from 40 to 600 Da. The spectrum of the components were compared with the database of a spectrum of known components stored in the GC-MS NIST (2008) library.

3.14.2 FOURIER TRANSFORM INFRARED SPECTROSCOPY (FT-IR)

Fourier Transform Infrared (FT-IR) Spectrometer was used to find the functional groups present in the chemical component. FT-IR spectra were recorded with a Perkin Elmer-Spectrum RXI Spectrometer equipped with a Mullard I-alanine doped triglycinesulfate (DTGS) detector. The spectrometer was continuously purged with dry nitrogen to eliminate atmospheric water vapor and carbon dioxide. The sample was scanned at 25 ± 1 °Cin the

4000-400 cm-1 spectral range. To improve the signal to noise ratio for each spectrum, 100 interferograms with a spectral resolution of ±4 cm-1 were averaged. The spectrum was analyzed using Origin 6.1 software.

3.14.3 UV SPECTROSCOPY

The purified compound of *C. albidum* Fraction1 (CA1) was dissolved in methanol and the spectrum was measured by using Double beam UV-VIS Spectrophotometer (200-800 nm), SL210, Elico, India. Methanol without sample was used as a blank.

3.14.4 NUCLEAR MAGNETIC RESONANCE (NMR) ANALYSIS

Nuclear Magnetic Resonance (NMR) analysis of isolated compounds was carried out in Vellore Institute of Technology- Sophisticated Instrumentation facility (VIT-SIF) Lab, School of Advanced Science (SAS), Chemistry division. Proton (1H) and carbon (13C) NMR of isolated compounds were assessed by Bruker Advance III 500 MHz A V 500. Ten mg of the compound was dissolved in 1 ml CDCl3 and pipette into NMR tube using Pasteur pipette with glass wool for filtration. The filtration was necessary to remove undissolved materials and dust from the sample. This could influence to change the clarity and shape of spectra. All the spectra results were compared with published information on previous literature and elucidate the structures of the isolated compounds.

3.14.5 MASS SPECTROMETRY (MS)

The Mass spectrum of the purified compound were documented by an electron impact (ESI) mode at 70 EV. The source, probe and scanning temperatures, which were used in this study was 0-300°C.

3.15 DETERMINATION OF ANTIOXIDANT ACTIVITY OF ISOLATED COMPOUND

3.15.1 DPPH RADICAL SCAVENGING ASSAY (Raman, 2006)

The DPPH free radical scavenging activity of methanol extract of isolated compound CA1 was carried out according to the method of Raman, (2006). One ml of Plant extract of various concentrations (5- 25 µg/ml) was mixed with 1 ml of 0.1 mm DPPH solution in acetone. The reaction mixture was kept in dark at room temperature for 30 min. Absorbance was read at 517 nm in a spectrophotometer. Ascorbic acid was used as the standard reference. The percentage of radical scavenging activity was calculated as follows,

3.15.2 HYDROXYL RADICAL SCAVENGING ASSAY (Halliwell *et al.*, 1981)

$$\% \text{ of inhibition} = \frac{\text{control- sample}}{\text{control}} \times 100$$

Hydroxy % of inhibition was carried out by Deoxyribose method followed by H ... µM EDTA, 100 µM FeCl3, 1 mM ... CA1 compound at various concentrations (25-150 µg) and the final reaction volume of 2ml was made with potassium phosphate buffer (20 mM, pH 7.4). The above mixture was kept at 37°C for 60 min, then add 1 ml each of 2.8% TCA, 0.5% TBA and 0.025 M NaOH containing 0.02% BHA and reaction mixture was heated at 95°C in a water bath for 15 min. Finally, the reaction mixture was allowed to cool and the absorbance was recorded at 532 nm. The negative control without sample, which was considered as 100% deoxyribose oxidation. Ascorbic acid was taken as positive control.

$$\% \text{ of inhibition} = \frac{\text{control- sample}}{\text{control}} \times 100$$

3.15.3 SUPEROXIDE RADICAL SCAVENGING ASSAY (Gangwar *et al.*, 2014)

Super oxide radical scavenging capacity of CA1 compound was determined by the inhibition of formazan production of nitroblue tetrazolium (NBT) (Gangwar *et al.*, 2014). A test tube contains 3 ml of reaction mixture which includes 0.01 M phosphate buffer (pH 7.8), 60 μM riboflavin,130 mM methionine, 0.5 mM EDTA and 0.75mM NBT with 0.5 ml of CA1 compound. The reaction mixture was kept in fluorescent light for 6 minutes and the absorbance value was measured at 560 nm. The nonenzymatic phenazine methosulfatenicotinamide adenine dinucleotide (PMS-NADH) system generates superoxide radicals, which reduce NBT to purple formazan. Ascorbic acid was taken as positive control.

3.15.4 NITRIC OXIDE RADICAL SCAVENGING ACTIVITY (Garrat, 1964)

Nitric oxide (NO) radical scavenging activity was evaluated by the Griess IlIosvoy reaction method followed by Garrat, (1964). The decompose of sodium nitroprusside in aqueous solution at physiological pH (7.2) which is spontaneously generating the nitric oxide. NO reacts with oxygen to produce stable products like nitrate and nitrite in aerobic conditions. The quantities of which can be determined using Griess reagent. Scavengers of nitric oxide compete with oxygen leading to reduced production of nitrite ions. In an experiment, sodium nitroprusside (10 mM) in phosphate-buffered saline was mixed with different concentrations (20- 120 µg/ml) of CA1 and ascorbic acid and incubated at 30°C for 2 hrs. The reaction mixture is added with 0.5 ml of Griess reagent (1% sulfanilamide, 0.1% N-(1-naphthyl) ethylenediamine dihydrochloride and 2% H_3PO_4), which is resulted in the formation of chromophore during diazotization of nitrite with sulfanilamide and consequent coupling with Naphthylethylenediamine dihydrochloride. The absorbance of chromophore formation was measured at 550nm.

$$\% \text{ of inhibition} = \frac{\text{control- sample}}{\text{control}} \times 100$$

3.16 *IN VITRO* ANTI-INFLAMMATORY ACTIVITY OF ISOLATED COMPOUND CA1 ON RAW 264.7 MACROPHAGES

3.16.1 CHEMICALS

Lipopolysaccharide (LPS), Phenol free Dulbecco's modified Eagle medium (DMEM), MTT, Dimethyl sulphoxide (DMSO), phosphate buffer saline (PBS), and antibiotic-antimycotic solution (100U penicillin, 100µg streptomycin, and 0.25µg amphotericin B per ml) were purchased from Sigma-Aldrich. Foetal bovine serum (FBS) was purchased from GIBCO/BRL Invitrogen.

3.16.2 CELL CULTURE

Macrophage RAW 264.7 cells were obtained from the NCCS, Pune with Passage no 9. Cells were cultured in phenol red-free DMEM supplemented with 100units/ml penicillin, 100µg/ml streptomycin, and 10% heat-inactivated FBS at 37°C with 5% CO_2. Cells were washed with DMEM medium and detached with 0.25% trypsin-EDTA. The cells were resuspended in DMEM medium at a density of 2 x 10^6 cells/ml.

3.16.3 CYTOTOXICITY ASSAY (González-Chávez *et al.*, 2017)

MTT assay, which is based on the conversion of MTT to MTT-formazan by mitochondrial enzymes present in the live cells, was used to assess the cytotoxicity of the crude extract and its respective fraction. The cells were plated in 96-well plates at a density of 5×10^3 cells/well. After 24h, the cells were washed with fresh medium and were treated with control medium or medium supplemented with different concentrations (5 – 320µg/ml) of crude extract and fraction. After incubation for 24h, cells were rewashed, 100µl of MTT solution (5mg/ml) was added, and the cells were incubated for an additional 4 h. Finally, 100µl of dimethyl sulphoxide (DMSO) was added to solubilize the formazan crystals. The amount of formazan present in each well was determined by measuring the absorbance of each well at 540nm with a hybrid microplate reader. Relative cell viability was determined by measuring the amount of MTT converted into formazan crystals.

3.16.4 MEASUREMENT OF NITRIC OXIDE PRODUCTION

RAW 264.7 cells (2×10^5cells/well) were seeded onto 96-well plates with DMEM without phenol red. The cells were allowed to adhere overnight and then were pre-treated with different concentrations (5–320µg/ml) of fraction for 1h. Cellular nitric oxide (NO) production was stimulated by adding 1µg/ml (final concentration) of lipopolysaccharide (LPS). LPS-stimulated cells were incubated for 4h. After incubation, Griess reagent (1% sulfanilamide, 5% phosphoric acid, and 0.1% N-(1-naphthyl) ethylenediamine hydrochloride) was used to determine NO production. Briefly, 50µl of supernatant from the test culture was mixed with 50µl of 1% (w/v) sulphanilic acid in 5% (v/v) phosphoric acid in a 96-well plate, followed by incubation for 10 min at room temperature. After that 50µl 0.1% (w/v) N-1-naphthylethylenediamine HCl in distilled water was added and incubated for 10 min at room temperature. After 15min of incubation at room temperature, the absorbance was measured at 550nm with a hybrid microplate reader. The percentage inhibition of NO production was calculated (Green *et al.*, 1982)

3.16.5 RNA ISOLATION AND Q - PCR ANALYSIS

RAW macrophages were treated with 27.5, 55 and 110µg/ml of a fraction with 1µg/ml of LPS and incubated for 24h.Total RNA was isolated using TRIzol reagent (*Invitro*gen) according to the manufacturer's protocol, and 2µg of RNA was used for complementary DNA synthesis using M-MLV reverse transcriptase (Promega, Madison, Wisconsin, USA). Quantitative real-time polymerase chain reaction (q-PCR) was performed in an ABI 7500 Real-Time System with SYBR Green PCR Master Mix (Takara). Reactions were initiated with an initial incubation at $50°C$ for two minutes and $94°C$ for 10 min, followed by40 cycles of $94°C$ for 5s, $60°C$ for 15s, and $72°C$ for 10s. The relative gene expression levels were calculated using the $2-\Delta\Delta Ct$ method. The specific primer sequences used were given below:

iNOS:	Forward:	5′-ATGTCCGAAGCAAACATCAC-3′
	Reverse:	5′-TAATGTCCAGGAAGTAGGTG-3′
COX-2:	Forward:	5′-CAGCAAATCCTTGCTGTTCC-3′
	Reverse:	5′-TGGGCAAAGAATGCAAACATC-3′
IL-6:	Forward:	5'-TCCAAACATCCTCCCCCAAAT-3'
	Reverse:	5'-AAAGGCGGCTTAGTTAGATCCC-3'
IL-1β	Forward:	5′-ATGGCAACTGTTCCTGAACTCAACT-3′
	Reverse:	5′-TTTCCTTTCTTAGATATGGACAGGAC-3′
TNF-α	Forward:	5′-ATGAGCACAGAAAGCATGATC-3′
	Reverse:	5′-TACAGGCTT GTCACTCGAATT-3′
IL -10	Forward:	5'-AGGCGCTGTCATCGATTTCT-3'

Reverse: 5'-ATGGCCTTGTAGACACCTTGG-3'

β-actin was used as an internal reference gene between different samples.

3.17 DETERMINATION OF *IN VITRO* ANTICANCER ACTIVITY OF CA1 USING HUMAN CERVICAL CANCER (HELA) CELL LINES

Minimum essential low glucose medium (MEM), Dimethyl sulfoxide (DMSO), penicillin, streptomycin, trypsin-EDTA were purchased from Lonza. MTT (3-(4,5-dimethylthiazol-2-yl)-2,5-diphenyltetrazolium bromide), Fetal bovine serum (FBS) was obtained from *In vitro* gen technologies. All other chemicals were of analytical grade.

3.17.1 CELL PREPARATION AND CULTURING

The HeLa human cervical cancer cell line was procured from NCCS with the passage number of 14. Cells were maintained in Minimum Essential Media (MEM) with low glucose supplemented with 10% Fetal Bovine Serum (FBS), with 100units/ml penicillin and 100µg/ml streptomycin. Cells were cultured in a humidified atmosphere with 5% CO_2 at 37°C. Cells were grown in $25cm^2$ culture flask and after a few passages, cells were seeded for experiments. The experiments were done at 70 to 80% confluence. Upon reaching confluence, cells were detached using 0.25% Trypsin-EDTA solution.

3.17.2 CELL PROLIFERATION ASSAY OR MTT ASSAY (Safadi *et al.*, 2003)

Cytotoxicity of the test drugs (Crude extract and fraction) was assessed by MTT assay (Safadi *et al.*, 2003). Cells were plated in 96-well plate at a concentration of 5×10^4 cells/well 24h after plating. After 24h of cell incubation, the medium was replaced with 100µl medium containing test drugs (Crude extract and fraction) at different concentrations 5 – 320 µg/well and incubated for 24h. Untreated cells served as control and received only 0.1% DMSO in which the test drugs were prepared. At the end of the treatment period, media from control, test drugs-treated cells were discarded and 50 µl of MTT (5mg/ml PBS) was added to each well. Cells were then incubated for 4h at 37°C in a CO_2 incubator. MTT was then discarded and the colored crystals produced formazan were dissolved in 150µl of DMSO and mixed effectively by pipetting up and down. Spectrophotometrical absorbance of the purple-blue formazan dye was measured using an ELISA reader (BIORAD) at 570nm. The optical density of each sample was compared with control optical density and graphs were plotted.

3.17.3 ETHIDIUM BROMIDE/ACRIDINE ORANGE (DUAL STAINING) (Gohel *et al.*, 1999)

Ethidium bromide/acridine orange staining was carried out by the method of Gohel *et al.*, 1999. HeLa cells were plated at a density of 5×10^4 in 12-well plates. They were allowed to grow at 37°C in a humidified CO_2 incubator until they were 70–80% confluent. Then cells were treated with 54μg/ml and 108μg/ml of the fraction (selected based on the IC_{50} concentration) for 24h. The culture medium was aspirated from each well and cells were gently rinsed twice with PBS at room temperature. Then equal volumes of cells from control and drug-treated were mixed with 100μl of dye mixture (1:1) of ethidium bromide and acridine orange) and viewed immediately under Optika view inverted fluorescence microscope (Ti series) at 10x magnification. A minimum of 200 cells was counted in each sample at 5 different fields. The percentage of apoptotic cells was determined by

$$\% \text{ of apoptotic cells} = \frac{\text{total number of apoptotic cells}}{\text{total number of cells counted}} \times 100$$

3.17.4 DETERMINATION OF INTRACELLULAR REACTIVE OXYGEN SPECIES (ROS) GENERATION (Akimoto *et al.*, 2015)

The formation of ROS was measured using a non - fluorescentprobe, 2, 7-diacetyl dichlorofluorescein (DCFH-DA) (Akimoto *et al.*, 2015). The non-fluorescent probe penetrates into the intracellular matrix of cells, where it isoxidized by Reactive oxygen species (ROS) and form fluorescent dichlorofluorescein (DCF). The production of ROS was estimated in terms of % fluorescence intensity in control and fraction 54μg/ml and 108 μg/ml treated HeLa cells. Briefly, an aliquot of the scraped cells 5×10^6 cells/ml was made up to a final volume of 2 ml in normal PBS (pH 7.4). Then, 1ml aliquot of cells was taken to which 100 μL DCFH-DA (10 μM) was added and incubated at 37°C for 30 min. Fluorescent measurements were made with excitation and emission filters were set at 485±10 nm and 530±10 nm respectively (Perkin Elmer Multimode reader). All initial fluorescent values (time

0) were found to differ from each other by less than 5%. Results were expressed as a percentage; an increase in fluorescence was calculated using the formula $[(Ft30-Ft0)/(Ft0\times100)]$, and the fluorescence intensities at 0 and 30 min were measured. Stained cells from each group were examined and imaged under the Optika view fluorescence inverted microscope.

3.17.5 FLOW CYTOMETRY

To investigate the effect of the plant fraction on cell cycle distribution, HeLa cells (1×10^6 cells/ml) were treated with 54µg/ml & 108µg/ml of the fraction for 24h. The treated cells were harvested, washed with phosphate buffer saline (PBS) and fixed in 75% ethanol at 4°C overnight. After washing twice with cold PBS, cells were suspended in PBS containing 40µg/ml Propidium iodide (PI) and 0.1mg/ml RNase A followed by shaking at37°C for 30min. The stained cells were analyzed with a flow cytometer (Becton-Dickinson San Jose, CA, USA) and the data were consequently calculated using Win MDI 2.9 software (TSRI, La Jolla, CA, USA) (Tu *et al.*, 2004).

3.17.6 GENE EXPRESSION ANALYSIS – REAL-TIME PCR

The HeLa cells were cultured in six-well plates and exposed to 54µg/ml and 108µg/ml of plant fraction for 24 hours. At the end of the exposure, total RNA was extracted by Trizol reagent according to the standard protocol. Isolated RNA was quantified using a Nano drop and cDNA was synthesized using a commercial kit (high cDNA, Applied Biosystem). Quantitative real-time PCR (qPCR) was performed in AbiPrismTM 7700 sequence detection system (Applied Biosystems). Gene-specific primers for Bax, Bcl2, Cytochrome C, Caspase 3 and Caspase 9 were used. β – actin was used as housekeeping control. The change in fluorescence of SYBR Green dye in every cycle was monitored, and the threshold cycle (ct) above background for each reaction was calculated. Results are expressed as fold change in gene expression with respect to the controls (Laura, 2005).

3.18 STATISTICAL ANALYSIS

Sufficient triplicates in experiments were carried out to avoid error and statistical calculation were made. Data obtained from the experiments were expressed as Mean ± SEM. The Statistical analysis of the difference between the groups was evaluated by Dunnett's following one way ANOVA Posthoc comparisons in Graph pad Prism 7.0 software version. p<0.001, p<0.01 and p<0.05 were considered to be statistically significant.

RESULTS

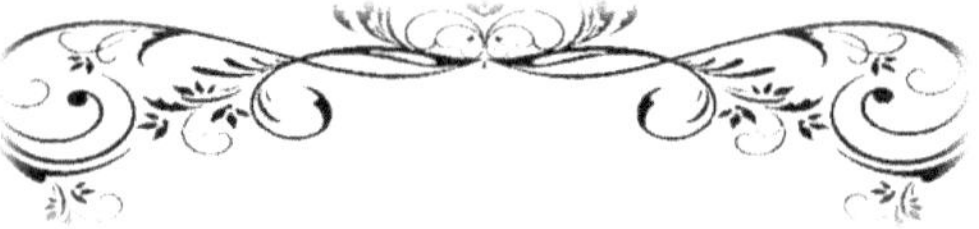

CHAPTER- IV

RESULTS

4.1 ETHNOBOTANICAL STUDY

The ethnobotanical survey of Thiruvadisoolam village of Kancheepuram District, Tamil Nadu, India made in the present study observed with total of 54 plant species from 46 Genera, belonging to 35 families, which are found medicinally important. The higher number of plant species recorded in the order of dominance as Apocynaceae (7 genera), Leguminosae (5 genera), Phyllanthaceae (4 genera) and Lamiaceae (3 genera). The number of other plant species was found less than two which were belonging to various families indicated in **Table 2 and Figure 15**. It was also observed from the survey that the plant leaves (24%) were the widely used plant part for various human ailments, followed by seeds and whole plants which are also used in remarkable numbers *i.e.* 10-15% (**Figure 16**).

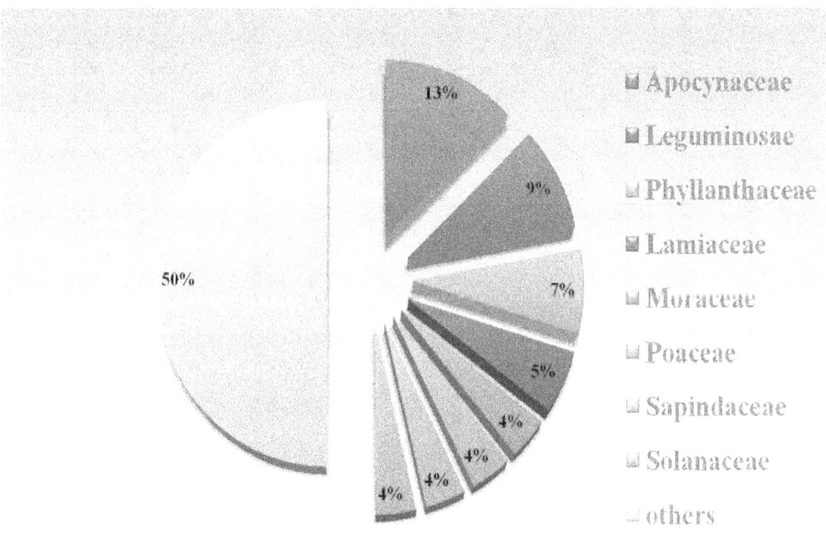

Fig 15: Enumeration of family counts (%) of medicinal plants collected from Thiruvadisolam

TABLE 2: LIST OF FOLKLORE MEDICINAL PLANTS DATA COLLECTED IN THE STUDY AREA

Botanical name	Genera	Family	Local name	Parts Used	Ethno medicinal Uses
Aristida setacea Retz.	*Aristida*	Poaceae	Thodappapullu	Root	Antidote and Antitoxic
Aristolochia bractiata. Lam.	*Aristolochia*	Aristolochiaceae	Aduthindapalai	Leaves	Asthuma
Artabotrys hexapetalus (L.f.) Bhandari	*Artabotrys*	Annonaceae	Manoranjitham	Leaves root	Chinese folk remedy for malaria
Asclepias curassavica Linn.	*Asclepias*	Apocynaceae	Aathuarali	Root	Antidote and Antitoxic
Asparagus racemosus Willd.	*Asparagus*	Asparagaceae	Thannirmuttansedi/ Jannikodi/Neermuthi	Root/Leaf	Roots tonic, aphrodisiac induce immunity and Demulscent
Atalanti amonophylla DC.	*Atalanti*	Rutaceae	Kattuelumichai	Leaves, root and bark	Antiallergic and antitoxic
Azadirachta indica A.Juss.	*Azadirachta*	Meliaceae	Vembu	Whole plant	Antimicrobial and Antitoxic
Bambus abambos (L.) Voss.	*Bambus*	Poaceae	Moongil	Leaves	Young shoots and leaves used to cure anti allergic stomach problem.
Brassica juncea (L.)Czern.	*Brassica*	Brassicaceae	Kadugu	Seed	Ache lumbago and rheumatism useful amenorrhea.
Caesalpinia pulcherrima (L.) sw.	*Caesalpinia*	Leguminosae	Mailkondrai	Seed	Reduces Tooth ache
Caesalpinia jayabo M. Gomez	*Caesalpinia*	Leguminosae	Kalakkai	Leaves, fruits and seed.	Febrifuge and antiperiotic.
Calophyllum inopyyllum L.	*Calophyllum*	Clusiaceae	Punnai	Seed	Oil from seed used in skin disease medicines, vermicide

Dryand.					
Cardiospermum halicacabum L.	*Cardiospermum*	Sapindaceae	Mudakkatham	Whole plant	Anti arthritic, tonic
Carissa carandas L.	*Carissa*	Apocynaceae	Kara pazam	Flower	Cure white Filmy eyes
Carissa spinarum L.	*Carissa*	Apocynaceae	Kala pazam	Flower	Cures, Ophthalmic disorders
Carmona retusa (Vahl) Masamune	*Carmona*	Boraginaceae	Kuruvingi	Fruits	Cough, colic, diarrhea and dysentery
Cassia auriculata (L.) Roxb.	*Cassia*	Caesalpiniaceae	Avaram poo	Flowers	Antidiabetic, blood purifier.
Coleus forskohlii (Willd.) Briq.	*Coleus*	Lamiaceae	Maruthuvacoorgam	Whole plant	Leaf diuretic, cures respiratory disease asthma disorder
Combretum albidum G.Don.	*Combretum*	Combretaceae	Karlankodi, Jalukodi	Fruits, steam, bark and Leaves	Diarrhea and dysentery.
Datura metel L.	*Datura*	Solanaceae	Oomathai	Leaves	Juice of leaves and few drops in poured into ear to treat earache.
Dodonaea viscose (L.) Jacq.	*Dodonaea*	Sapindaceae	Kattuarali	Leaves	Pain killer
Erythrina variegata L.	*Erythrina*	Gentianaceae	Kalyanamurungai	Leaves park	Cures Liver trouble joint pain, dysentery.
Euphorbia hirta L	*Euphorbia*	Euphorbiaceae	Amman pacharice	Whole plant	human bacterial pathogens
Ficus benghalensis L.	*Ficus*	Moraceae	Aalamaram	Latex	The milk exudates of the plant is applied externally in rheumatic complaints.
Ficusre ligiosa L.	*Ficusre*	Moraceae	Arasamaram	Leaves	The dried leaf of arasu is powdered mixed with water and takes normally to relief from budding pain.
Gisekia pharnaceoides L.	*Gisekia*	Aizoaceae	Nagamalli	Leaf	Antiseptic

Gmelina asiatica L.	*Gmelina*	Verbenaceae	Nilakumizh/ Mulkumizh	Leaf	Antiulcer, wound healing
Guizotia abyssinica (L.f.) Cass.	*Guizotia*	Compositae	Malaiellu	Seeds	Seed oil is used reduce the weight of the body, stomachic oil used treatment of rheumatism, regulates heart function.
Gymnema sylvestre (Retz.) R.Br. ex Sm.	*Gymnema*	Apocynaceae	Sirukurinjan	Leaves	Antidiabetic
Hemidesmus indicus (L.) R.Br.exSchult.	*Hemidesmus*	Apocynaceae	Nannari	Root	Tonic, diaphoretic diuretic, coolant
Hibiscus rosa-sinesis L.	*Hibiscus*	Malvaceae	Semparuthi	Leaves ,flower	Hair tonic, hair wash. Menorrhagia
Kirganelia reticulata. (poir) Baill.	*Kirganelia*	Euphorbiaceae	Karunelli	Fruit, root & Leaf	Diuretic, alterative and for cooling effect and also used for smallpox.
Mangifera indica L.	*Mangifera*	Anacardiaceae	Maamaram	Seeds	Leucorrhagia menorrhagia.
Marsileaqua drifolia L.	*Marsileaqua*	Marsileaceae	Aarakeerai	Leaves	Leaf juice Cures Snakebite and applied abscesses.
Ocimum tenuiflorum L.	*Ocimum*	Lamiaceae	Tulasi	Whole plant	Cure cold ,cough
*Ocimum basilicum*L.	*Ocimum*	Lamianceae	Thiruneetrupachilai	Leaves	Antiseptic
Phyllanthus emblica L.	*Phyllanthus*	Euphorbiaceae	Peru Nelli	Fruit &root mixed	Hepatictonic and hepato protective
Phyllanthus amarus Schumach.&Thonn.	*Phyllanthus*	Phyllanthaceae	Nelli	Fruit &root mixed	Hepatic tonic hepato protectic
Phyllanthu sniruri L.	*Phyllanthus*	Phyllanthaceae	Keezha nelli	Whole plant	Hepatoprotective liver tonic
Plumbago zeylanica L.	*Plumbago*	Plumbaginaceae	Sithiramoolam	Root	Antitoxic Febrifuge(Fever

					reducing)
Santalum album L.	*Santalum*	Santalaceae	Santhana maram	Leaf Bark	Cures Urinary tract infection &anti diabetes
Saraca indica L.	*Saraca*	Fabaceae	Ashokamaram	Leaf	Central Nervous System
Scoparia dulcis L.	*Scoparia*	Plantaginaceae	Sakkarainilavembu	Whole plant	Ant diabetic, Emetic
Senna alata (L.) Roxb.	*Senna*	Leguminosae	Vandukolli	Leaves	Cures Fungal infection and skin cures
Sesamum indicum L.	*Sesamum*	Pedaliaceae	Ellusedi	Seeds, Leaves	Demulcent, coolant and laxative
Solanum virginianum L.	*Solanum*	Solanaceae	Kandankathirikai	Leaves	Dried leaf powder boiled with castor oil the mixture is taken orally treat all type of skin diseases.
Stachytarpheta indica (L.) Vahl.	*Stachytarpheta*	Verbenaceae	Seemai Naayuruvi	Whole plant	Leucorrhoea
Strychnos nux –vomica L.	*Strychnos*	Loganiaceae	Yetti	Seeds	Antitoxic, Antidote
Syzygium cumini (L.) Skeels.	*Syzygium*	Myrtaceae	Navalmaram	Fruit Seeds	Tonic , Ant diabetic cures
Wrightia tinctoria R.Br	*Wrightia*	Apocynaceae	Veppalai	Latex	Latex applied externally to get relief from anythorn pricked in head to leg.
Zingiber officinale Roscoe	*Zingiber*	Zingiberaceae	Inghi	Whole plant	Antiarthritic, antiulcer, anti allergic. Rhizome juice is used to cure skin infection like eczemaring worm.
Ziziphus jujube Mill.	*Ziziphus*	Rhamnaceae	Elandi	Fruit	Blood purifier

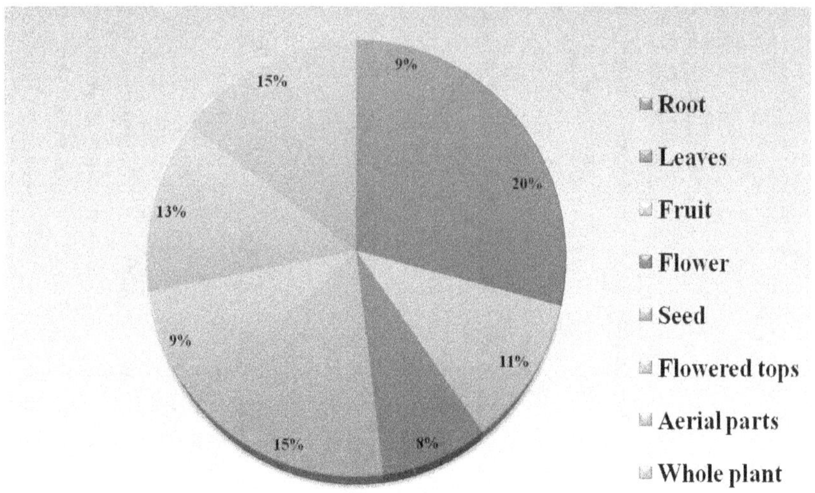

Fig 16: Percentage details of different parts of the medicinal plants used for various ailments

From the ethnobotanical survey it was observed that the tribal and local herbal users have been using several plants to cure numerous diseases including fever, skin diseases, anticancer, diabetes, vomiting, wounds, anticonvulsant, antipyretic, purgative, jaundice, liver diseases, leprosy, bronchitis, earache, increase sperm count in men, cardiotonic, urinary troubles, blood purification, increase the memory, carminative, antiepileptic, syphilis indigestion, antidote, anemia, chest pain, burns, dog bites, ulcer, aphrodisiac, anti-asthmatic, scabies, sedative, reduce body heat, bitter tonic, diuretic, uterus disorders, fever, facial paralysis, anti-fertility, antiseptic, toothache, dysentery, fits, colic pain, prevention of white discharge in women, healing borne fracture, anti-inflammatory, amoebic dysentery, refrigerant, diaphoretic, brain tonic, hemorrhagic enteritis, kidney problems, etc. Different plant parts are used in various preparations like infusions, decoctions, fumigation, maceration, powder, cream, bath, tablets and the majority of the plants were in the form of powder.

In the present assessment, 44 native herbalists from the study area were interviewed, and their details were presented in **Table 3**. Men (74%) dominate the practice of traditional medicine due to the cultural traditions of the region, where women are not encouraged to work. The age group of herbalists varied from 31 to 40 (41%) and over 60 years is a very low-frequency group (6%). About one-third of herbalists are illiterate (34%).

All the plant species were well-known to the informants interviewed and were perfectly recognized by their vernacular names. This means that the medicinal properties of some of these species can seriously be considered for further ethnopharmacological analysis since they are widely practiced by many people and they have been using for a long time. The majority of the medicinal plants were present in all the collection sites, but few species were seen in the selected area only. Despite the herbalist knew most of the medicinal plants available there, all species could not be always found in all areas. Based on the information from villagers and literature collection, the most medicinally valuable and abundant plants such as *Z. officinale*, *S. nux-vomica*, *G. Asiatica*, *E. hirta*, *P. emblica*, *C. acriculata*, *C. retusa*, *C. spinarum*, *C. albidum* and *K. reticulata* were selected for further studies.

TABLE 3: LITERACY RATE OF THE STUDY AREA

Literacy Rate / Age Frequency	Total Count	Illiterate		Primary		Secondary		Academic	
		Male	Female	Male	Female	Male	Female	Male	Female
21 to 30	09	1	1	1	1	2	0	2	1
31 to 40	16	0	0	2	1	3	2	7	1
41 to 50	15	2	3	3	2	2	2	1	0
51 to 60	04	2	1	0	0	1	0	0	0
Total	44	5	5	6	4	8	4	10	2

Literacy status data collected from the informants in the survey area.

4.2 PRELIMINARY SCREENING FOR PHYTOCHEMICALS

4.2.1 QUALITATIVE PHYTOCHEMICAL ANALYSIS OF PLANT PARTS

The methanolic plant extracts of selected 10 species of plants were tested for the presence of various phytoconstituents such as phenols, alkaloids, flavonoids, glycosides, saponins, terpenoids, proteins, tannins, steroids and reducing sugars by performing different qualitative tests and their results were presented in **Table 4 & Figure 17**. The details of phytoconstituents present in individual species were as given below.

Z. officinale

The methanolic extract of *Z. officinale* shows the presence of phenols, alkaloids, flavonoids, glycosides, terpenoids, proteins, tannins and steroids. The saponins and reducing sugars are absent in the methanolic extract of *Z. Officinale* (**Table 4**).

S. nux-vomica

The plant extracts show positive reports on phenols, flavonoids, terpenoids, proteins, tannins and steroids and negative results for glycosides, alkaloids, saponins and reducing sugars (**Table 4**).

G. asiatica

The phytochemicals such as phenols, alkaloids, flavonoids, glycosides, saponins, terpenoids, proteins, and tannins were present in methanolic extract of *G. asiatica* at the same time the steroids and reducing sugars were showing negative results (**Table 4**).

C. auriculata

The methanolic extract of *C. auriculata* was found with the presence of phenols, alkaloids, flavonoids, glycosides, saponins, terpenoids, proteins, tannins and reducing sugars, except steroids, which is negative results (**Table 4**).

P. emblica

The phytochemicals such as phenols, alkaloids, flavonoids, glycosides, saponins, terpenoids, proteins, and tannins shows positive results in methanolic extract of *P. emblica* at the same time the steroids and reducing sugars were negative results (**Table 4**).

E. hirta

The plant *E. hirta* contains five components such as phenols, flavonoids, saponins, terpenoids and tannins whereas glycosides, alkaloids, proteins, steroids and reducing sugars were absent in the extract (**Table 4**).

C. retusa

From all the 10 selected plants the methanolic extract of *C. retusa* shows the presence of less number of phytochemicals such as phenols, flavonoids, glycosides, and tannins. While the phytochemicals like alkaloids, proteins, saponins, terpenoids, steroids and reducing sugars were found absent in the qualitative test (**Table 4**).

C. spinarum

The methanolic extract of *C. spinarum* shows the presence of phenols, alkaloids, flavonoids, glycosides, saponins, terpenoids, proteins and tannins, whereas the steroids and the absence of reducing sugars (**Table 4**).

C. albidum

C. albidum shows the presence of 7 groups of phytoconstituents such as alkaloids, phenols, glycosides, terpenoids, flavonoids, tannins and steroids. However, Phytoconstituents such as reducing sugars, saponins and proteins were absent (**Table 4**).

K. reticulata

Alkaloids, phenols, glycosides, tannins, saponins, and proteins were present in *K. Reticulate* methanolic extract and phytochemicals such as terpenoids, flavonoids, reducing sugars and steroids were found absent (**Table 4**).

TABLE 4: PRELIMINARY PHYTOCHEMICAL ANALYSIS OF SELECTED MEDICINAL PLANTS

Phytochemicals	Z. officinale	S. nux-vomica	G. asiatica	E. hirta	P. emblica	C. acriculata	C. retusa	C. spinarum	C. albidum	K. reticulata
Alkaloids	P	A	P	A	P	P	A	P	P	P
Phenols	P	P	P	P	P	P	P	P	P	P
Glycosides	P	A	P	A	P	P	P	P	P	P
Terpenoids	P	P	P	P	P	P	A	P	P	A
Flavonoids	P	P	P	P	P	P	P	P	P	A
Tannins	P	P	P	P	P	P	P	P	P	P
Reducing Sugars	A	A	A	A	A	P	A	A	A	A
Saponins	A	A	P	P	P	P	A	P	A	P
Proteins	P	P	P	A	P	P	A	P	A	P
Steroids	P	P	A	A	A	A	A	A	P	A

A-Absent; P-Present

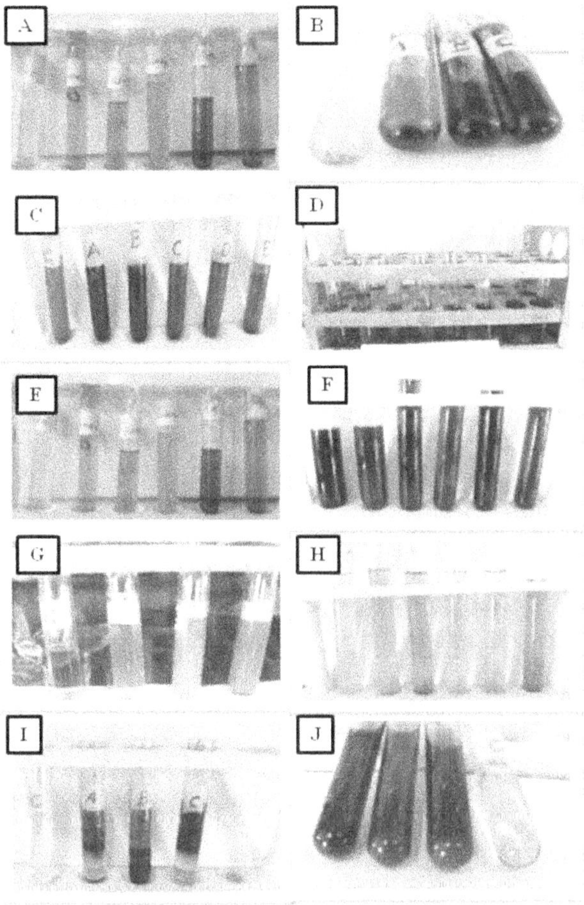

Figure 17. Qualitative phytochemical screening of selected medicinal plants A-Tannin B- Terpenoids C- Steroids D-Glycosides E-Protein F-Phenol G-Saponins H-Flavonoids I- Alkaloids J- Reducing sugars

4.2.2 QUANTITATIVE PHYTOCHEMICAL ANALYSIS

4.2.2.1 TOTAL PHENOLIC CONTENT

The total phenolic content of the methanolic extract of 10 selected medicinal plants was measured using the Folin-Ciocalteu method and the results were indicated in **Table 5**. The highest phenolic content was found in *C. albidum* (212.1 mg GAE/g) and the lowest phenolic content was found in *S. nux-vomica* (12.56 mg GAE/g). The quantity of phenol content present in other plant species in the decreasing order are as in *P. emblica* (152.55 mg GAE/g), *Z. officinale* (119.75 mg GAE/g), *K. reticulata* (117.59 mg GAE/g), *G. asiatica* (60.49 mg GAE/g), *C. auriculata* (28.43 mg GAE/g), *C. retusa* (27.11 mg GAE/g), *C. spinarum* (19.2 mg GAE/g) and *E. hirta* (14.22 mg GAE/g), respectively **(Figure 18).**

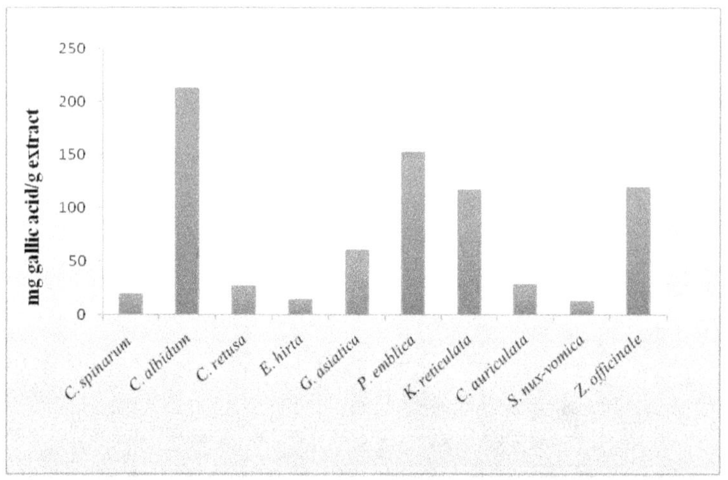

Figure 18 : Total phenolic content of methanolic extract of different medicinal plants

4.2.2.2 TOTAL FLAVONOID CONTENT

As presented in **Table 5**, the total flavonoid content of different plant methanolic extracts was examined by using the aluminium chloride method and the results were expressed as mg QE/g of the extract. The flavonoid content of methanolic extracts was varied greatly from 8.26 to 143.06 mg QE/g **Figure 19**. The methanolic extract of *C. albidum* showed highest flavonoid content (143.06 mg QE/g), followed by *Z. officinale* (128.11mg QE/g), *E. hirta* (125.71 mg QE/g), *G. Asiatica* (108.42 mg QE/g), *S. nux-vomica* (88.64 mg QE/g), *K. reticulata* (84.86 mg QE/g), *C. retusa* (36.51 mg QE/g), *C. auriculata* (18.99 mg QE/g) and *P. emblica* (13.04 mg QE/g), while *C. spinarum* showed the lowest flavonoid content as 8.26 mg QE/g, respectively.

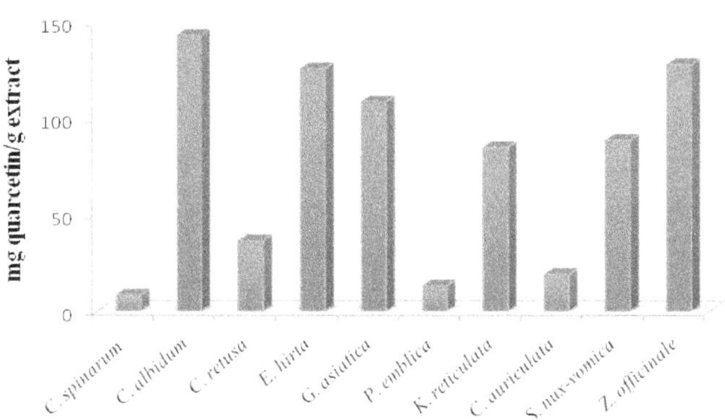

Figure 19: Total flavonoid content of methanolic extract of different medicinal plants

TABLE 5: QUANTITATIVE PHYTOCHEMICAL ANALYSIS OF SELECTED MEDICINAL PLANTS

Methanolic plant extracts	Phenols (mg gallic acid/g extract)	Flavonoids (mg quarcetin/g extract)
C. spinarum	19.2	8.26
C. albidum	212.1	143.06
C. retusa	27.11	36.51
E. hirta	14.22	125.71
G. asiatica	60.49	108.42
P. emblica	152.55	13.04
K. reticulate	117.59	84.86
C. auriculata	28.43	18.99
S. nux-vomica	12.56	88.64
Z. officinale	119.75	128.11

4.3 ANTIBACTERIAL ACTIVITY OF PLANT EXTRACTS

Antibacterial activity screening of 10 different plant methanolic extracts against two gram positive bacteria such as *M. luteus*, *B. subtilis* and two gram negative bacteria such as *S. typhi and P. mirabilis* were carried out in comparison with standard antibiotic streptomycin. Among the 10 medicinally important plants selected for antibacterial activity, *C. albidum* exhibited highest inhibition zone against the bacteria such as *S. typhi* (14 mm), *M. luteus* (22 mm) and *P. mirabilis* (18 mm) and *E. hirta* showed highest activity against *B. subtilis* (18 mm). The lowest antibacterial activity against *S. typhi* was 7 mm showed by *Z. officinale*, *C. retusa* and *S. nux-vomica*; *M. luteus* was 5 mm by *G. asiatica*; *P. mirabilis* was 6 mm by *S. nux-vomica* and *B. subtilis* was 7mm by *C. retusa* and *S. nux-vomica*. The results for antibacterial activity test is presented in **Table 6, Figure 20 & Figure 21**.

TABLE 6: ANTIMICROBIAL ACTIVITY OF METHANOLIC EXTRACT OF SELECTED MEDICINAL PLANTS

Plant Extracts	Bacterial Growth (Zone of inhibition in mm)			
	S. typhii	*M. lutens*	*P. mirabilis*	*B. subtilis*
Z. officinale	7	7	9	10
C. carandas	9	6	7	11
E. hirta	14	6	13	18
S. nux-vomica	7	10	6	7
P. embilica	13	19	7	9
G. asiatica	13	5	10	8
C. auriculata	8	9	8	12
C. retusa	7	13	8	7
K. reticulata	8	12	10	13
C. albidum	14	22	18	13
streptomycin	23	30	28	24

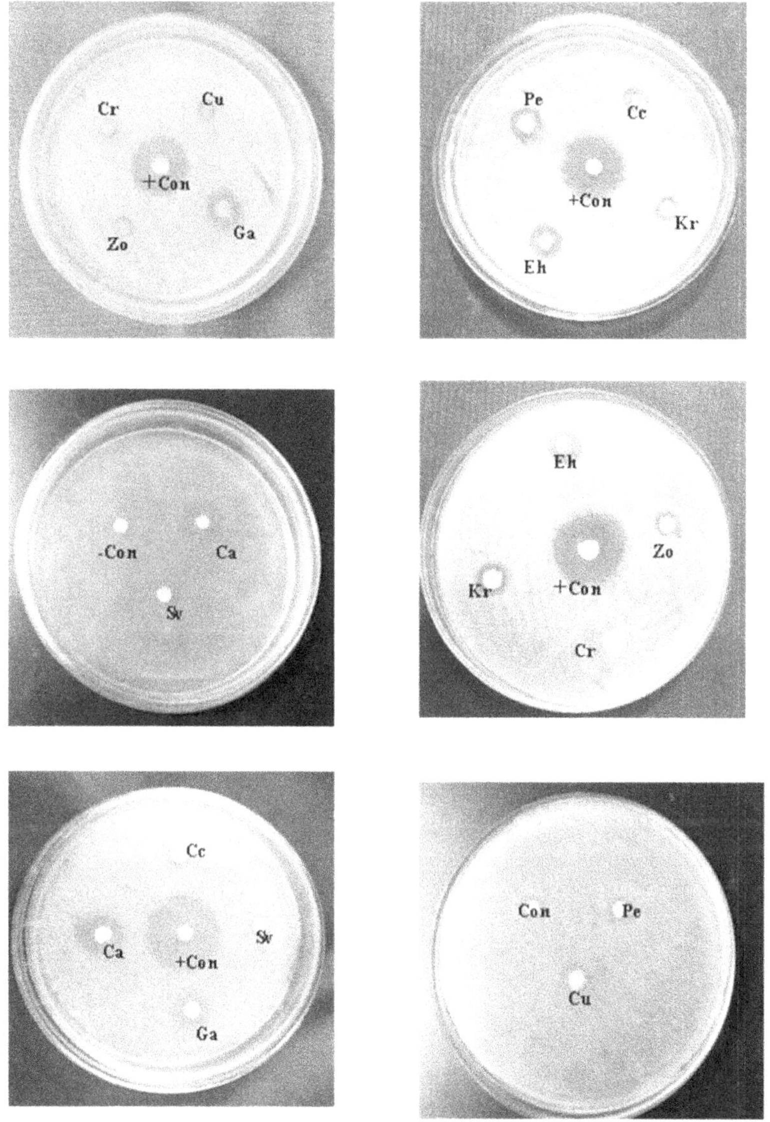

Figure 20. Effect of plant methanolic extracts against gram negative Bacteria *Salmonella typhii and Proteus mirabilis*

Zo- *Z. officinale,* **Cc-** *C. spinarum,* **Eh-** *E. hirta,* **Sv-** *S. nux-vomica,* **Pe-** *P. embilica,* **Ga-** *G. asiatica,* **Cu-** *S. auriculata,* **Cr-** *C. retusa,* **Kr-** *K. reticulata,* **Ca-** *C. albidum,* **+Con-** Streptomycin, **-Con -** Methanol

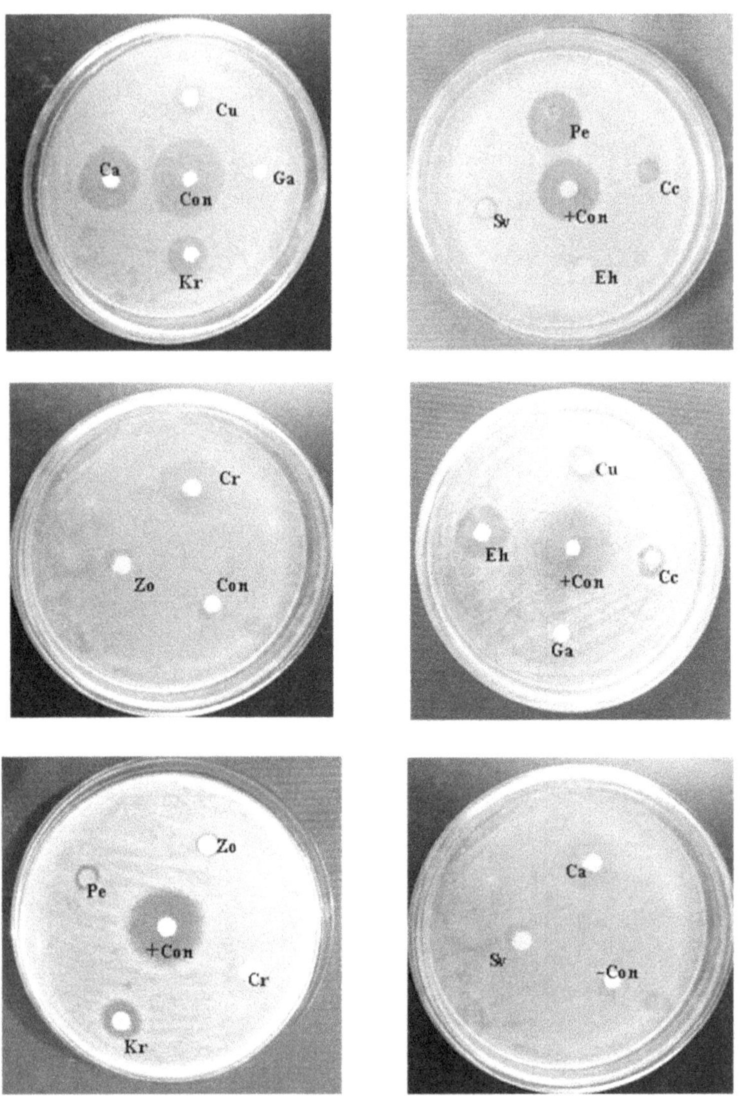

Figure 21. Effect of plant methanolic extracts against gram negative Bacteria *Micrococcus luteus and Bacillus subtilis*
Zo- *Z. officinale*, **Cc-** *C. spinarum*, **Eh-** *E. hirta*, **Sv-** *S. nux-vomica*, **Pe-** *P. embilica*, **Ga-** *G. asiatica*, **Cu-** *S. auriculata*, **Cr-** *C. retusa*, **Kr-** *K. reticulata*, **Ca-** *C. albidum*, **+Con-** Streptomycin, **-Con** - Methanol

4.4 EVALUATION OF ANTIOXIDANT ACTIVITY

4.4.1 PHOSPHOMOLYBDENUM REDUCTION ASSAY

The total antioxidant capacity of methanolic plant extracts of selected medicinal plants was observed by the Phosphomolybdenum reduction assay. The methanolic extracts show that the absorbance of Phosphomolybdenum reduction at 320 µg/ml were from 0.08 to 1.36, where *C. spinarum* (0.08), *C. retusa* (0.12), *S. nux-vomica* (0.29), *G. asiatica* (0.35), *C. auriculata* (0.62), *E. hirta* (0.78), *P. emblica* (0.85), *Z. officinale* (1.08), *K. reticulata* (1.1) and *C. albidum* (1.36), respectively. Therefore the methanolic extract of *C. albidum* plant shows highest absorbance values when compared to other plant extracts, which indicates significant leaf of antioxidant activity and the results are presented in **Table 7 & Figure 22**.

4.4.2 DETERMINATION OF DPPH RADICAL SCAVENGING ACTIVITY

The methanolic crude extracts of 10 plants were tested for it antioxidant activity and the highest percentage of radical scavenging activity was observed in *C. albidum* (65.94 %) followed by *Z. Officinale* (59.348 %), *C. auriculata* (58.42 %), *P. emblica* (57.77 %), *C. retusa* (55.29 %), *K. reticulata* (53.25 %), *C. spinarum* (51.92 %), *S. nux-vomica* (50.97 %), *G. asiatica* (50.76 %) and *E. hirta* (45.283 %), respectively at the concentration of 320 µg/ml (**Table 8 & Figure 23**). The 50% inhibition concentration of plant extracts including *C. albidum*, *Z. officinale*, *C. auriculata*, *P. emblica*, *C. retusa*, *K. reticulata*, *C. spinarum*, *S. nux-vomica* and *G. asiatica* was 147.74 µg/ml, 149.15 µg/ml, 273.83 µg/ml, 276.94 µg/ml, 289.38 µg/ml, 300.43 µg/ml, 308.16 µg/ml, 313.88 µg/ml and 315.15 µg/ml, whereas *E. hirta* doesn't show the IC_{50} value.

4.4.3. DETERMINATION OF FERRIC REDUCING POWER ASSAY

The reducing power activity of above 10 selected medicinal plants was determined and is shown in **Table 9**. The results showed that a significant dose-dependent reducing activity at various concentrations, ranging between 10 µg/mL and 320 µg/mL was exhibited by the extracts. The reducing power were in the order of following as *C. retusa= E. hirta >* *C. auriculata > G. asiatica > S. nux-vomica > P. emblica > K. reticulata> C. spinarum > Z. officinale > C. albidum* (**Figure 24**). All the above extracts exhibited lower reducing power when compared to standard ascorbic acid.

TABLE 7: DETERMINATION OF THE ANTIOXIDANT ACTIVITY OF SELECTED MEDICINAL PLANTS BY PHOSPHOMOLYBDENUM ASSAY

Plant extracts	Absorbance value					
	10 (µg/ml)	20 (µg/ml)	40 (µg/ml)	80(µg/ml)	160(µg/ml)	320(µg/ml)
C. albidum	0.36 ± 0.02	0.58 ± 0.04	0.73 ± 0.05	1.07 ± 0.07	1.24 ± 0.08	1.36 ± 0.09
C. auriculata	0.1 ± 0.007	0.19 ± 0.013	0.3 ± 0.021	0.37 ± 0.025	0.49 ± 0.034	0.62 ± 0.043
C. retusa	0.03 ± 0.002	0.05 ± 0.004	0.08 ± 0.005	0.1 ± 0.007	0.11 ± 0.008	0.12 ± 0.009
C. spinarum	0.01 ± 0.001	0.03 ± 0.002	0.05 ± 0.003	0.06 ± 0.004	0.07 ± 0.005	0.08 ± 0.006
E. hirta	0.25 ± 0.01	0.44 ± 0.03	0.5 ± 0.03	0.67 ± 0.04	0.7 ± 0.04	0.78 ± 0.05
G. asiatica	0.07 ± 0.005	0.17 ± 0.012	0.22 ± 0.015	0.31 ± 0.021	0.32 ± 0.022	0.35 ± 0.024
K. reticulata	0.28 ± 0.019	0.35 ± 0.024	0.5 ± 0.035	0.66 ± 0.046	0.88 ± 0.061	1.1 ± 0.077
P. emblica	0.32 ± 0.022	0.38 ± 0.026	0.48 ± 0.033	0.71 ± 0.049	0.76 ± 0.053	0.85 ± 0.06
S. nux-vomica	0.05 ± 0.003	0.11 ± 0.008	0.17 ± 0.012	0.22 ± 0.015	0.23 ± 0.016	0.29 ± 0.02
Z. officinale	0.22 ± 0.016	0.35 ± 0.024	0.6 ± 0.042	0.71 ± 0.049	0.97 ± 0.068	1.08 ± 0.075

Values were obtained in triplicate, expressed as the mean $\pm$ SD and found to be statistically significant at $p \leq 0.05$.

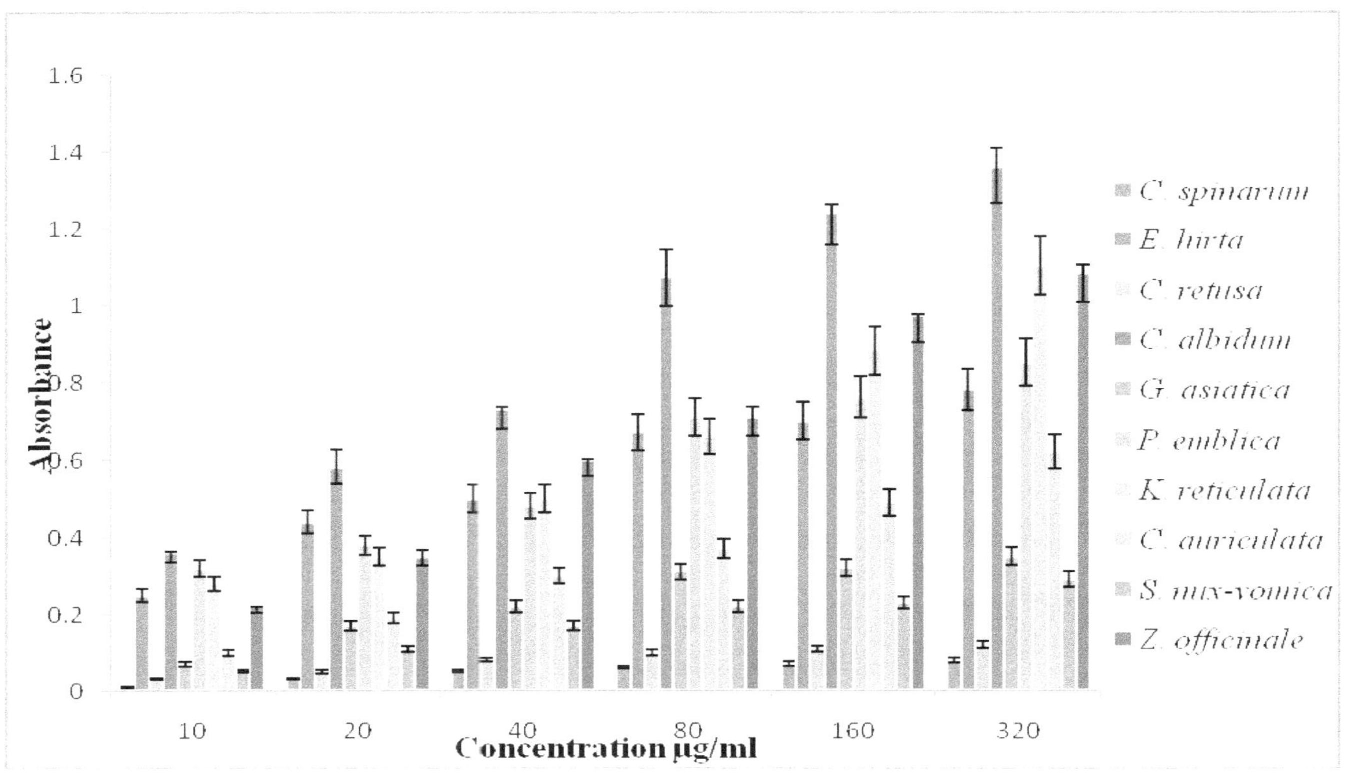

Figure 22: Determination of total antioxidant activity of selected medicinal plants

TABLE 8: DETERMINATION OF DPPH RADICAL SCAVENGING ACTIVITY OF SELECTED MEDICINAL PLANTS

Values were obtained in triplicate, expressed as the mean $\pm$ SD and found to be statistically significant at $p \leq 0.05$.

Plant extracts	Percentage of Inhibition					
	10 (µg/ml)	20 (µg/ml)	40 (µg/ml)	80 (µg/ml)	160 (µg/ml)	320 (µg/ml)
C. spinarum	7.057 ± 0.49	15.434 ± 1.08	21.434 ± 1.29	29.116 ± 2.03	41.838 ± 2.92	51.92 ± 3.63
C. albidum	16.334 ± 0.99	21.878 ± 1.39	31.027 ± 1.68	43.536 ± 2.53	54.146 ± 2.94	65.941 ± 3.21
C. retusa	14.168 ± 1.14	19.866 ± 1.53	24.127 ± 2.17	36.19 ± 2.69	42.094 ± 2.88	55.29 ± 3.56
E. hirta	5.974 ± 0.41	14.281 ± 0.99	21.698 ± 1.51	26.205 ± 1.83	37.133 ± 2.59	45.283 ± 3.16
G. asiatica	17.9 ± 1.25	22.1 ± 1.54	29.956 ± 2.09	36.313 ± 2.54	42.874 ± 3.00	50.768 ± 3.55
P. emblica	10.942 ± 0.76	18.071 ± 1.26	27.134 ± 1.89	40.213 ± 2.32	49.007 ± 2.92	57.774 ± 2.99
K. reticulate	6.966 ± 0.48	16.415 ± 1.14	24.219 ± 1.69	36.437 ± 2.55	43.837 ± 3.06	53.256 ± 3.77
C. auriculata	10.542 ± 0.73	18.175 ± 1.27	27.693 ± 1.93	33.046 ± 2.31	45.424 ± 2.89	58.429 ± 3.39
S. nux-vomica	13.183 ± 0.92	20.381 ± 1.42	26.315± 1.84	35.5 ± 2.48	42.776 ± 2.99	50.974 ± 3.49
Z. officinale	15.34 ± 0.37	26.976 ± 1.18	32.394 ± 1.56	46.96 ± 1.88	53.635 ± 2.56	59.348 ± 3.38

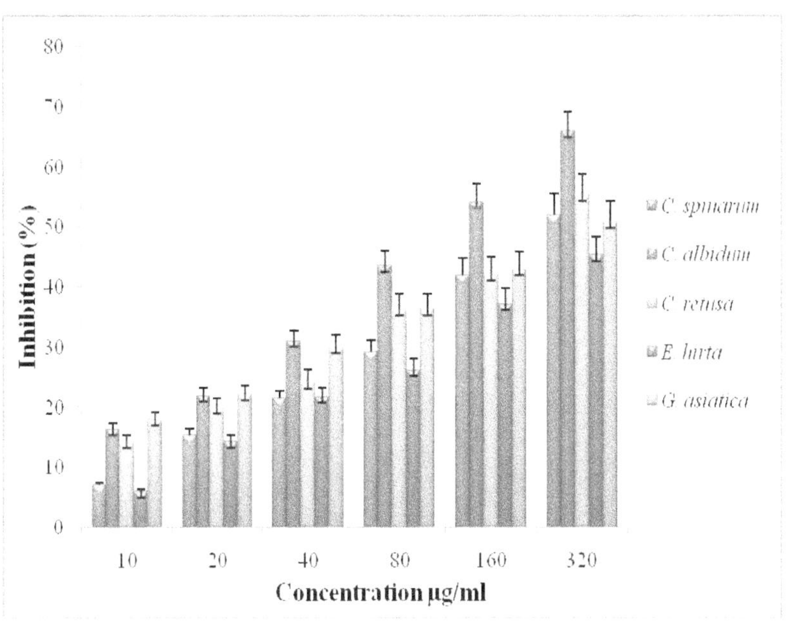

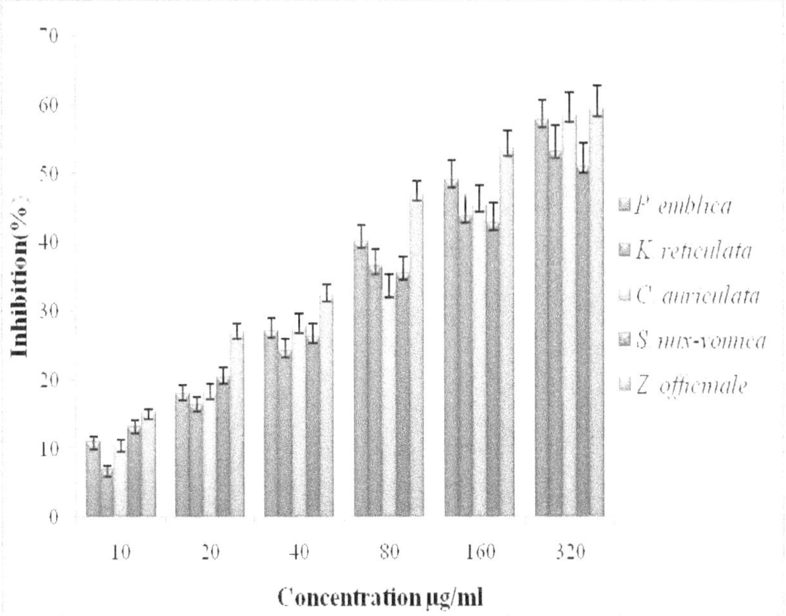

Figure 23. DPPH radical scavenging assay of selected medicinal plants

TABLE 9: DETERMINATION OF Fe^{3+} RRIC REDUCING POWER ASSAY OF SELECTED MEDICINAL PLANTS

Plant extracts	Absorbance value					
	10 (µg/ml)	20 (µg/ml)	40 (µg/ml)	80 (µg/ml)	160 (µg/ml)	320 (µg/ml)
C. spinarum	0.03 ± 0.0014	0.042 ± 0.002	0.072 ± 0.0035	0.118 ± 0.0058	0.148 ± 0.0072	0.237 ± 0.0411
K. reticulate	0.05 ± 0.0024	0.092 ± 0.0045	0.105 ± 0.0051	0.131 ± 0.0064	0.014 ± 0.0069	0.182 ± 0.009
C. retusa	0.019 ± 0.001	0.027 ± 0.0013	0.033 ± 0.0016	0.043 ± 0.0021	0.059 ± 0.0029	0.071 ± 0.0035
E. hirta	0.021 ± 0.001	0.023 ± 0.0011	0.038 ± 0.0018	0.047 ± 0.0023	0.061 ± 0.003	0.071 ± 0.0035
G. asiatica	0.028 ± 0.0013	0.039 ± 0.0019	0.046 ± 0.0022	0.07 ± 0.0034	0.1 ± 0.0049	0.111 ± 0.0054
P. emblica	0.054 ± 0.0026	0.069 ± 0.0034	0.085 ± 0.0042	0.124 ± 0.0061	0.166 ± 0.0081	0.178 ± 0.0088
C. albidum	0.106 ± 0.0052	0.212 ± 0.0104	0.227 ± 0.0112	0.276 ± 0.0136	0.299 ± 0.0148	0.41 ± 0.0202
C. auriculata	0.025 ± 0.0012	0.048 ± 0.023	0.066 ± 0.0032	0.077 ± 0.0038	0.091 ± 0.0045	0.096 ± 0.0047
S. nux-vomica	0.027 ± 0.001	0.037 ± 0.0018	0.067 ± 0.0033	0.077 ± 0.0038	0.135 ± 0.0066	0.144 ± 0.0071
Z. officinale	0.076 ± 0.0037	0.126 ± 0.0062	0.139 ± 0.0068	0.222 ± 0.0109	0.291 ± 0.0144	0.383 ± 0.0189

Values were obtained in triplicate, expressed as the mean ± SD and found to be statistically significant at $p \leq 0.05$.

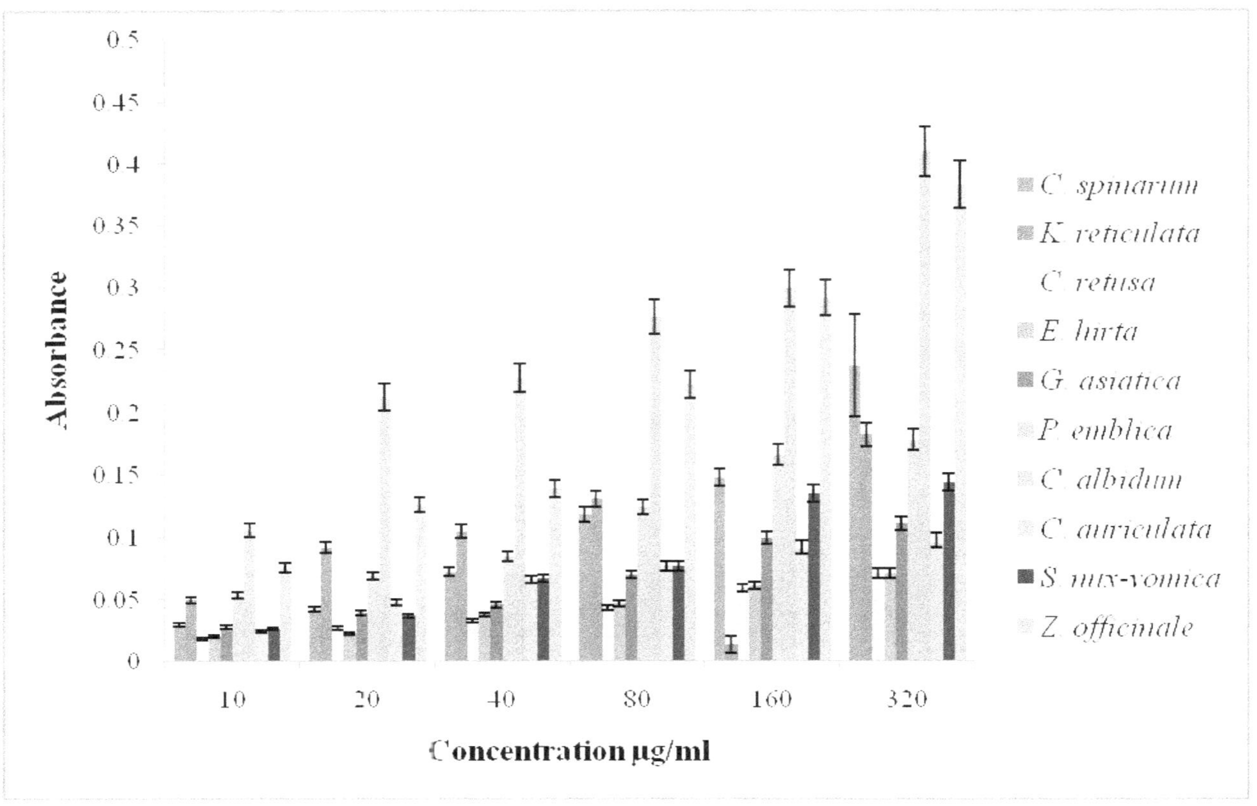

Figure 24. Fe^{3+} Reducing power assay of selected medicinal plants

4.5 PHARMOCOGNOSTIC STUDY

4.5.1 MACRO MORPHOLOGICAL DESCRIPTION

The leaf of *C. albidum* was simple and green in color. The shape of a leaf was oblong in size of 7-10 x 5-6.5 cm and the apex was acuminate with an entire margin. The surface was Papery with a petiole of 1-2 cm long, whereas as the taste was slightly bitter without specific odor. The results are indicated in **Table 10**.

TABLE 10: MACRO MORPHOLOGICAL DESCRIPTION

Characters	Observation
Leaf	Simple,
Shape	Oblong
Size	7-10 x 5-6.5 cm
Apex	Acuminate,
Margin	Entire
Base	Cuneate
Surface	Papery
Colour	Green
Taste	Slightly bitter
Odour	Not specific
Petiole	1 – 2 cm long

4.5.2 ANATOMY OF LEAF

The leaf has smooth and even surfaces; the midrib is slightly planoconvex and measures 750µm in thickness, the adaxial epidermis consist of small circular cells with thin cuticle. The abaxial epidermal cells are thin rectangular with fairly prominent cuticle. The ground tissues along with abaxial part of the midrib includes 3 -5 layers of small angular compact cells (**Figure 25.1**). The vascular system consists of a single prominent collateral vascular bundle which is broadly conical in outline.

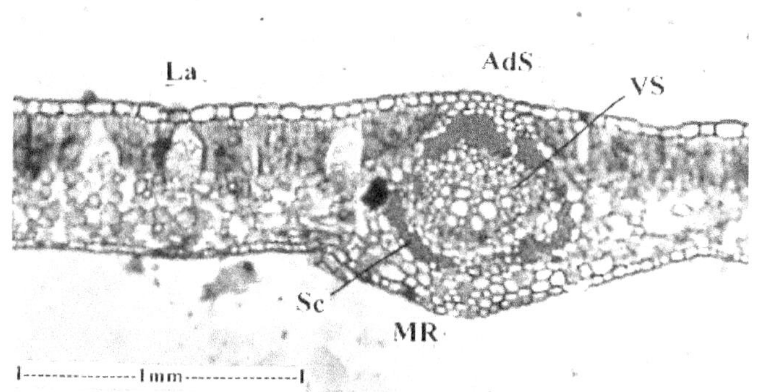

Figure 25.1. *C. albidum* **TS of Leaf though Midrib**

The vascular bundle is 90μm along the vertical plane and 120μm in horizontal plane. The vascular bundle is encircled with fairly thick sclearenchyma cells. The bundle consists of horizontal shallow arc of wide, circular, thick walled xylem elements, which are in air or wax vertical files. The protoxylem elements are in adaxial side. Phloem elements occurred in thin deep cup shaped are along with the lower part of xylem strands (**Figure 25.2**).

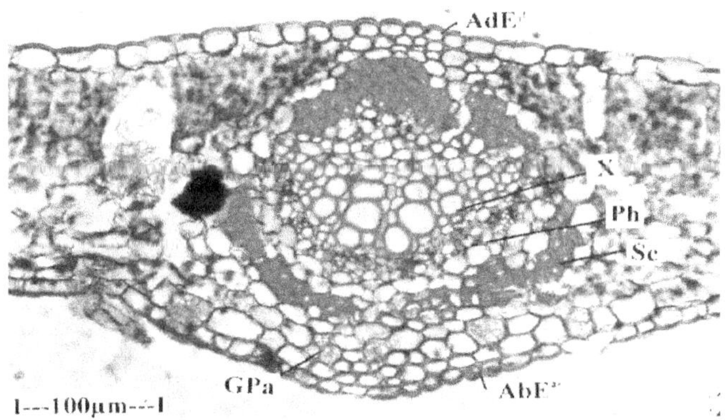

Figure 25.2. *C. albidum* **TS of Leaf Through Midrib Enlarged**

4.5.2.1 Lamina

The lamina is heteromorphic and bifacial with respect to the mesophyll tissues (**Figure 25.3**). The adaxial epidermal cells are elliptical or convex and have thick cuticle. The abaxial epidermis has small squarish thick walled cells. The mesophyll cells consist of adaxial horizontal band of vertically elongated pillar like palisade cells. Spongy mesophyll tissues includes about seven layers of spherical body arranged cells with wider air chambers. The lateral veins is prominent and well developed; it consists of adaxial mass of xylem elements and abaxial layer of phloem elements. The vascular bundles have prominent bowl shaped sclernchmatous abaxial and adaxial caps.

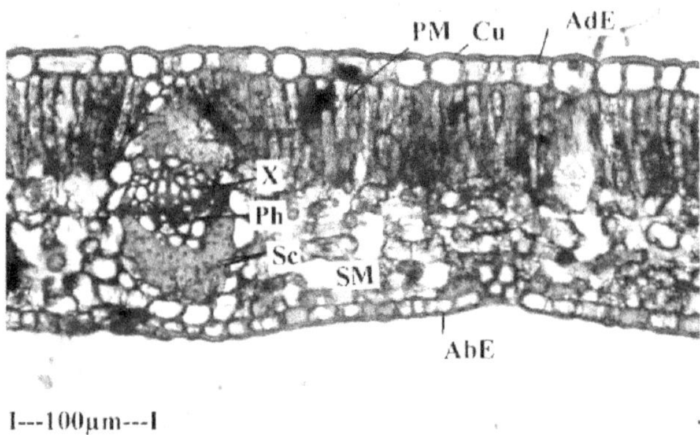

Figure 25.3. *C. albidum* **TS of Lamina**

4.5.2.2 Leaf Margin

The marginal part of the lamina becomes gradually tapering and forms a thick conical part. The epidermal cells of the marginal are smaller thick walled thickly cuticularized. The cells in the sub marginal part are wide thin walled and compact (**Figure 25.4**). The mesophyll tissues is an unchanged in the inner part of lamina.

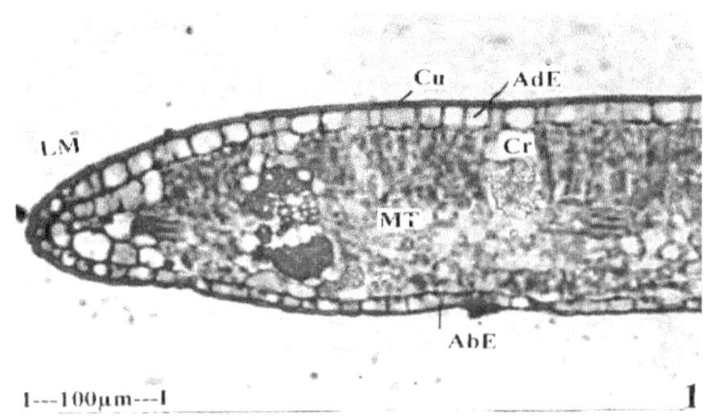

Figure 25.4. *C. albidum* **TS of Leaf Margin**

4.5.2.3 Crystals

Calcium oxalate crystals are common in the leaf tissues. The crystals are mainly druses or prismatic types. There is unique combination of the prismatic crystals and druses (**Figure 25.5**). The druses are normal in shape and size being spherical with minute spiny surfaces (**Figure 25.6**), this druses are located in the normal ordinary paranchymatous cells of the mesophyll tissues. Less frequently are seen druses which are quit large, vertically elongated and have larger spiny structures especially two longest and thick spines in two opposite poles (**Figure 25.7**). This type of crystals is located in the larger dilated mesophyll cells. Sometimes a prismatic crystals and druses type of crystals occur in a wide dilated cells which differs in shapes and sizes from neighboring cells Such cells are called crystalliferous idoblasts (**Figure 25.8**). The idioblast has a wide long prismatic crystalsover which a druses type of crystals are attached.

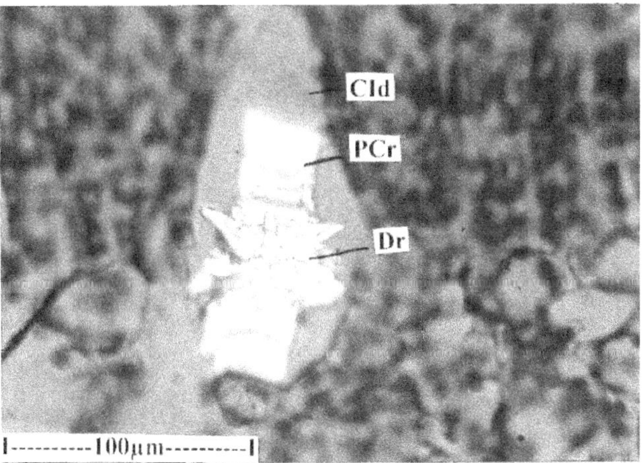

Figure 25.5. *C. albidum* TS of Leaf having Prismatic Crystal & Druses type of Crystal Ideo Blast

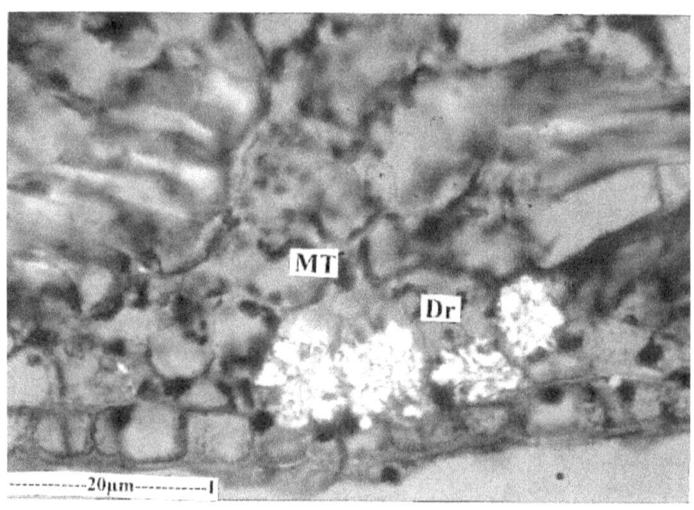

Figure 25.6. *C. albidum* Mesophyll Tissue with small normal type Of Druses

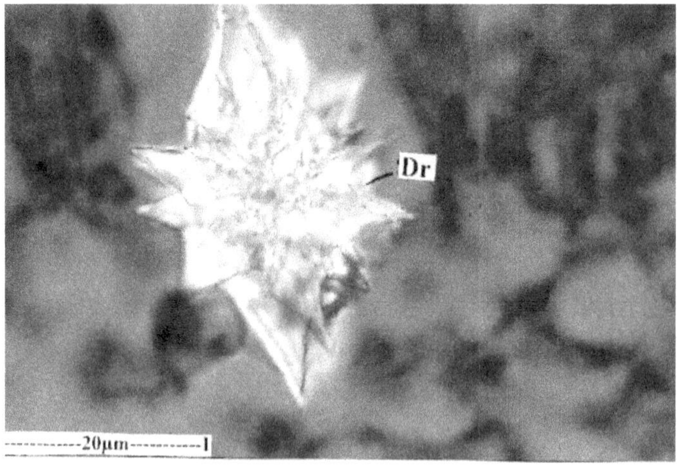

Figure 25.7. *C. albidum* Unusually large Druses type of crystal with long , spiny
outgrowth

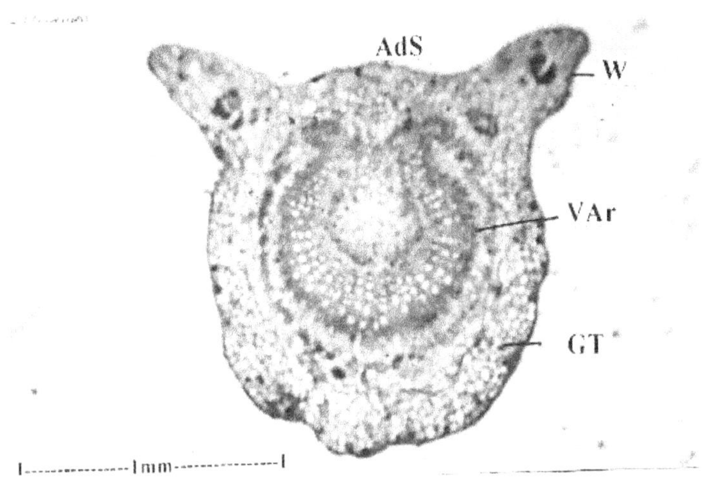

Figure 25.8. *C. albidum* **Mesophyll Tissue with small normal type of Druses**

4.5.2.4 Petiole

The petiole is circular in cross sectional view with two long thick wings on adaxial part of the petiole (**Figure 25.9**). The wings are lateral on the petiole. The petiole is 1.3mm in vertical and horizontal planes. The epidermal layer of the petiole is thin and the epidermal cells are small and circular in shape with thick walls. The ground tissues is paranchymatous and the cells are polygonal, thin walled and compact. The ground parenchyma cells are about eight layers (**Figure 25.10**).

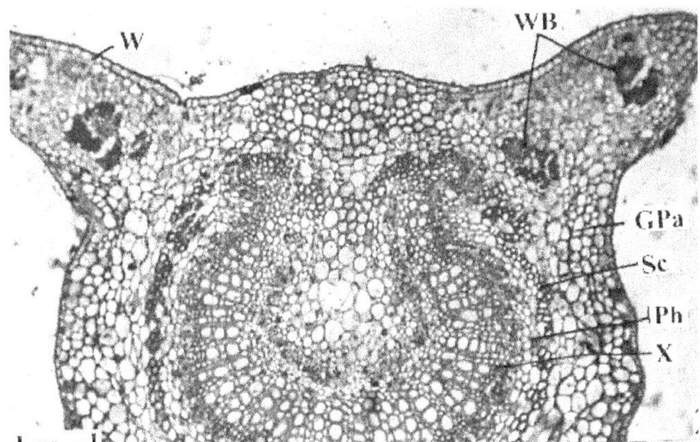

Figure 25.9. *C. albidum* **TS of Petiole Upper Sector**

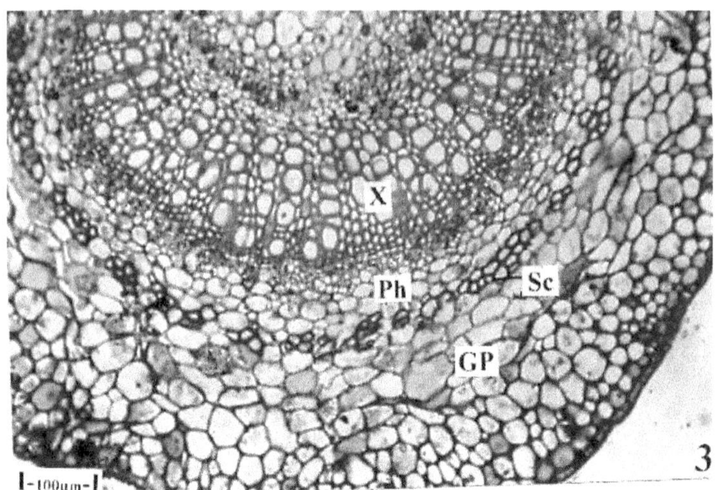

Figure 25.10. *C. albidum* Ts of Petiole Lower Sector

The vascular system of the petiole is large central in position and it is omega shaped in out line. The vascular strand has deep cup shaped main part and the two margins are curved out ward (**Figure 25.11**) and the vascular strand includes numerous vertical, parallel lines of xylem elements which are 6-8 cells in each lines. The xylem elements are wide, circular, thick walled and lignified. The protoxylem elements are dissected towards adaxial side. The cells in between the xylem lines are sclarenchymatous (**Figure 25.12**).

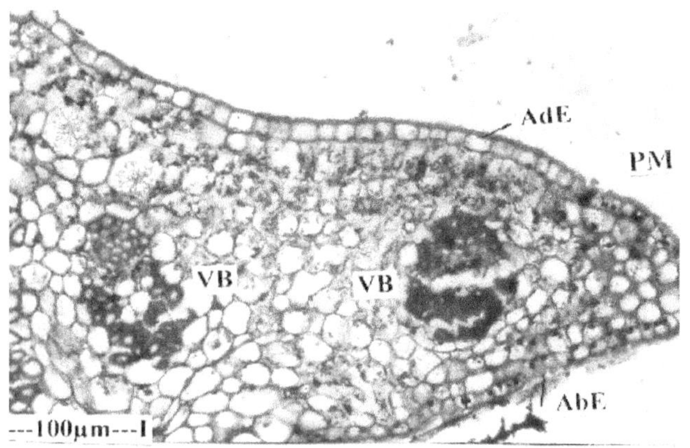

Figure 25.11. *C. albidum* TS of Petiole Margin

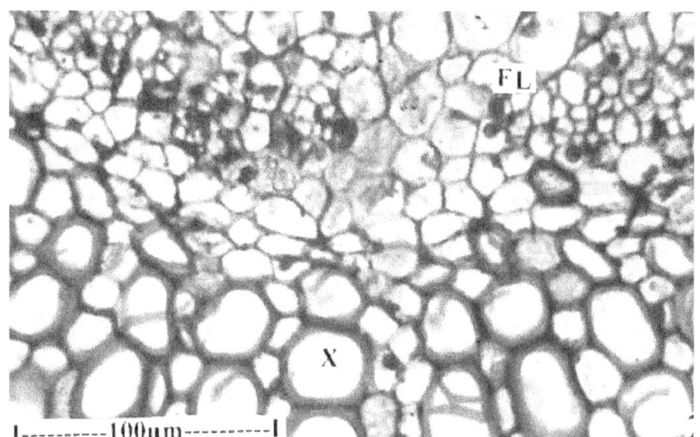

Figure 25.12. *C. albidum* **TS of Petiole middle part of the Vasculare Strand showing Xylem arc &Fibre layer inside the Xylem Strand**

Phloem occurs on the lower part of the xylem arc in discrete units of small masses (**Figure 25.13**). The phloem elements (sieve elements) are small in size and have shinking cell walls. Entire vascular strands are surrounded by thin continuous layer of sclarenchyma cells. The wings are thick and conical. The epidermal cells are wide and squarish with prominent cuticle (**Figure 25.13**). Beneath the epidermis a thin zone of chlorenchyma cells and the remaining tissue includes circular / angular parenchyma cells; there are two small vascular bundles. The bundles are collateral with a few wide xylem elements associated with phloem elements. The vascular bundles are covered partially by scleranchyma cells.

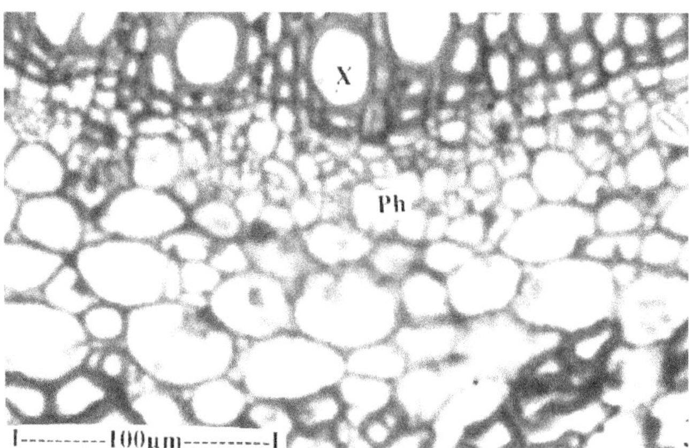

Figure 25.13. *C. albidum* **Ts of Petiole Showing Basal part of the Vascular Strand**

4.5.2.5 Leaf Epidermal cells

The epidermal tissues of lamina were studied from paradermal sections of the leaf. The adaxial epidermis of the lamina consists of polygonal, thick walled and the anticlinal walls are slightly waxy (**Figure 25.14**). The epidermis is apostomatic (without stomata).

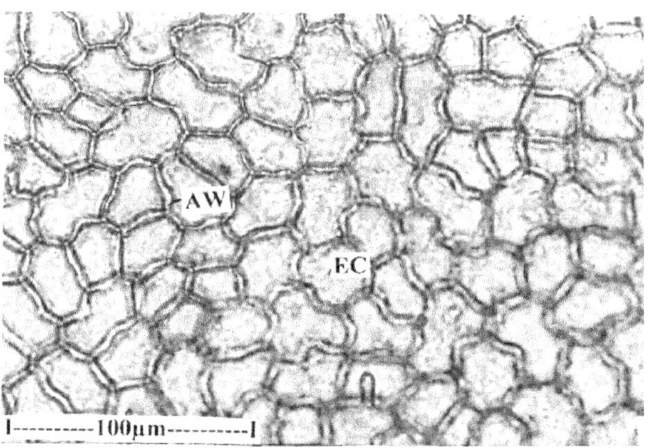

Figure 25.14. *C. albidum* **Surface view of Lamina showing Adaxial Epidermis**

The abaxial epidermis has smaller cells with thick straight anticlinal walls or slightly waxy walls (**Figure 20.15**). The abaxial epidermis is densely stomatiferous. The guard cells are broadly elliptical and measure 15x30µm in size. The cell walls of the guard cells at the end (polar) reign are thick (**Figure 25.16**). The stomata are surrounded by the three or four subsidiary cells, which are semicircular and are parallel to the long axis of the guard cells. Stomatal aperture is very narrow and slit like.

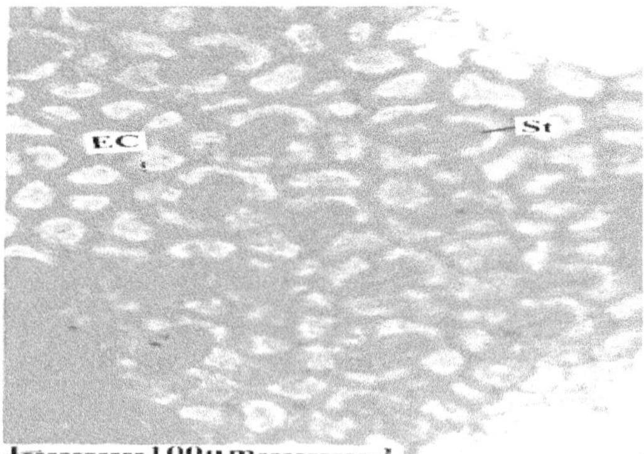

Figure 25.15. *C. albidum* **Abaxial epidermis surface view of Abaxial Epidermis shoeing Stomata**

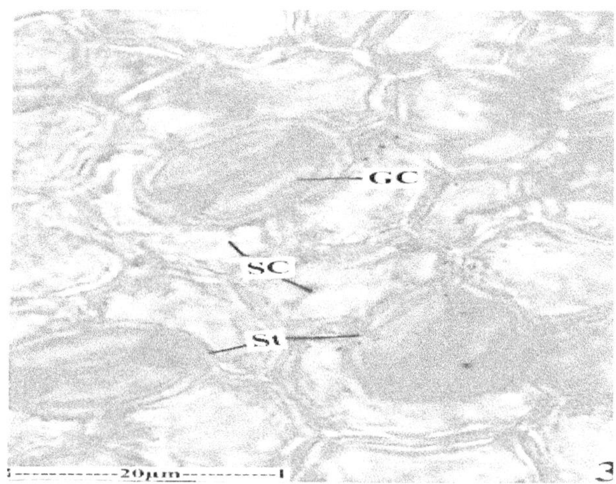

Figure 25.16. *C. albidum* **Stomata Enlarge**

4.5.2.6 Cicatrix

The epidermal tirchomes originate from modified epidermal cells. The trichome bearing epidermal cells are circular, thick walled and have narrow central cavity. The circular trichome bearing cells are called Cicatrix. The Cicatrix is surrounded by one or two circles of epidermal cells which are different in shape and size. Fine lines of cuticular striations are seen radiating from the Cicatrix and surrounding epidermal cells (**Figure 25.17**).

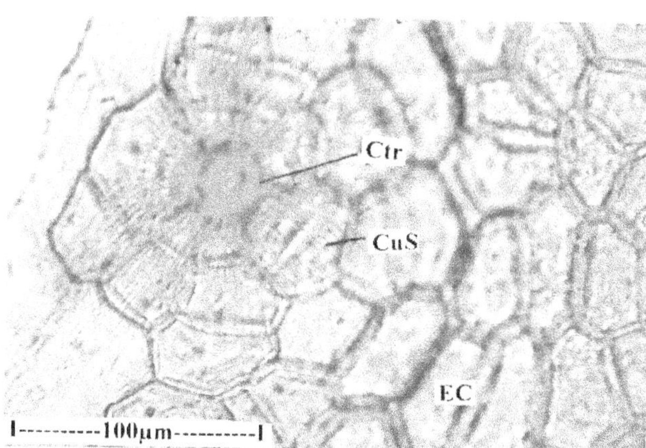

Figure 25.17. *C. albidum* **A Cicatrix with surrounding cells having radial cuticular stiriation**

4.5.2.7 Fibers

Thin librifrom fibers are often seen in isolated condition (**Figure 25.18**), these fibers are thin, long, and straight or curved, they thin walls and wide lumen or thick walls and narrow lumen, the fibers measures 400-850μm in length and 10μm in thick.

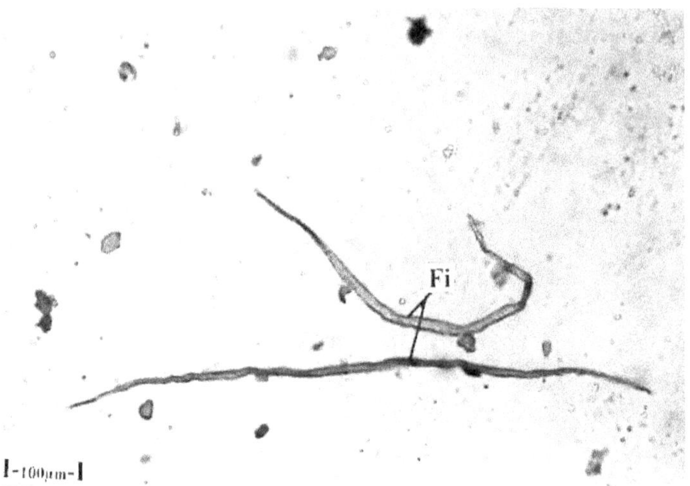

Figure 25.18. Libriform Fibres

4.5.3 PROXIMATE ANALYSIS

4.5.3.1 FLUORESCENCE ANALYSIS OF POWDER OF *C. ALBIDUM*

The *C. albidum* leaf powder was subjected to fluorescence analysis and demonstrated in **Table 11**. The leaf powder of *C. albidum* was observed in pale green color under daylight and emitted green color in UV light (254 nm). When the leaf powder was treated with concentrated HCl it shows green color in daylight and dark green under UV light. When treated in Concentrated HNO_3 and Picric acid shows green color in daylight, whereas in UV light yellowish color and the green color were observed, respectively. Treatment with 5% NaOH and Ferric chloride solution, results in brown and blue color in daylight, meanwhile, yellowish-green and black color was noticed in UV light. In daylight Pale, yellow and Orangish green was detected in conc. H_2SO_4 and ammonia treatment, whereas in UV light colorless and pale green were emitted, respectively.

TABLE 11: FLUORESCENCE ANALYSIS OF *C. ALBIDUM* LEAF POWDER WITH VARIOUS CHEMICAL REAGENTS.

Reagents	Color observed under Visible Light	Color observed under UV Light (254nm)
Powder as such	Pale Green	Green
Powder + Concentrated HCL	Green	Dark Green
Powder + Concentrated HNO3	Green	Yellowish Green
Powder + Concentrated H2SO4	Pale yellow	Colour less
Powder + 5% NaOH solution	Brown	Black
Powder + 5% Ferric chloride solution	Blue	Yellowish green
Powder + Picric acid	Green	Green
Powder + Ammonia	Orangish green	Pale green

4.5.3.2 PHYSICO-CHEMICAL PARAMETERS OF *C. ALBIDUM* LEAVES

The physiochemical parameters of *C.albidum* leaves were presented in **Table 12**. The moister content of *C.albidum* leaves was 13.7%. The ash value content is 8.1%, 0.24% and 5.84% for total ash, acid insoluble ash, and water-soluble ash, respectively. The extractive value of methanol (14.42 %) was higher when compared to aqueous extract (11.52), respectively.

TABLE 12: PHYSICO-CHEMICAL PARAMETERS OF *C. ALBIDUM* LEAVES

Parameter	Values (% w/w)
Moisture content	13.7% ±0.34
Ash Values	
Total Ash	8.1±0.70
Acid insoluble ash	0.24±0.37
Water soluble ash	5.84±0.24
Extractive Values	
Water soluble extractive	11.52±0.66
Methanol soluble extractive	14.42±0.81

Standard deviation (SD) = ±SD; Number of readings (N) =3

4.6 GC-MS ANALYSIS

The GC-MS analysis of a methanolic extract of *C. albidum* revealed to identify various compounds present. The various components present in the methanolic extract of *C. albidum* were detected based on the chromatogram of GC-MS which is shown in (**Figure 26**). The identified compounds are (i) Phenol, 2,4-bis-(1,1-dimethyl ethyl), (ii) Flavone, (iii) 6-methoxy flavone, (iv) palmitic acid, (v) oleic acid, (vi) Phytol, (vii) Coumarine, 3-[2-(1-methyl-2-imidazolylthio)-1-oxoethyl], (viii) 4-(benzyloxy)-4-(2,2-dimethyl-1,3-d dioxolane-4-yl)butanal, (ix) Stigmasterol, (x) Corynan-17-ol, 18,19-dihydro-10-methoxy-, acetate (ester), (xi) Pregna-4,6-diene-3,20-dione, 17-(acetyloxy)-6-methyl, (xii) Azafrin and (xiii) 6-Bromo-1,1,4,4,7-pentamethyl-1,2,3,4-tetrahydronaphthalene. The retention time, molecular weight and molecular formula were presented in **Table 13.**

4.7 THIN LAYER CHROMATOGRAPHY (TLC) OF *C. ALBIDUM* METHANOLIC LEAF EXTRACT

Thin-layer chromatography is uncomplicated, low cost and rapid technique used to separate and identify components in a complex mixture. TLC is exploited to separation and identification of components in a mixture by R_f value compared with standard compound R_f value. TLC of *C. albidum* methanolic extract was assessed in the hexane and ethyl acetate solvent system in the ratio of 9:1. The result shows 8 spots having different R_f values under UV light, daylight and iodine chamber (**Figure 27**). The R_f value of different compound spots are 0.107, 0.233, 0.326, 0.491, 0.629, 0.728, 0.823 and 0.974, respectively.

4.8 COLUMN CHROMATOGRAPHY (CC) OF *C. ALBIDUM* METHANOLIC LEAF EXTRACT

The methanol extract of *C. albidum* was subject to column chromatographed on a silica gel (100-200 mesh) column eluted with continuous hexane and ethyl acetate gradients. The solvent used was hexane with an increasing percentage of ethyl acetate, starting at 5, 10, 15, 20...100. Finally the column was washed with methanol (**Figure 28**). There are totally 14 fractions (each 500 ml) were eluted and the collected fractions were subjected to TLC. The active fraction CA1 was selected through antioxidant activity and it shows a single yellow spot on TLC.

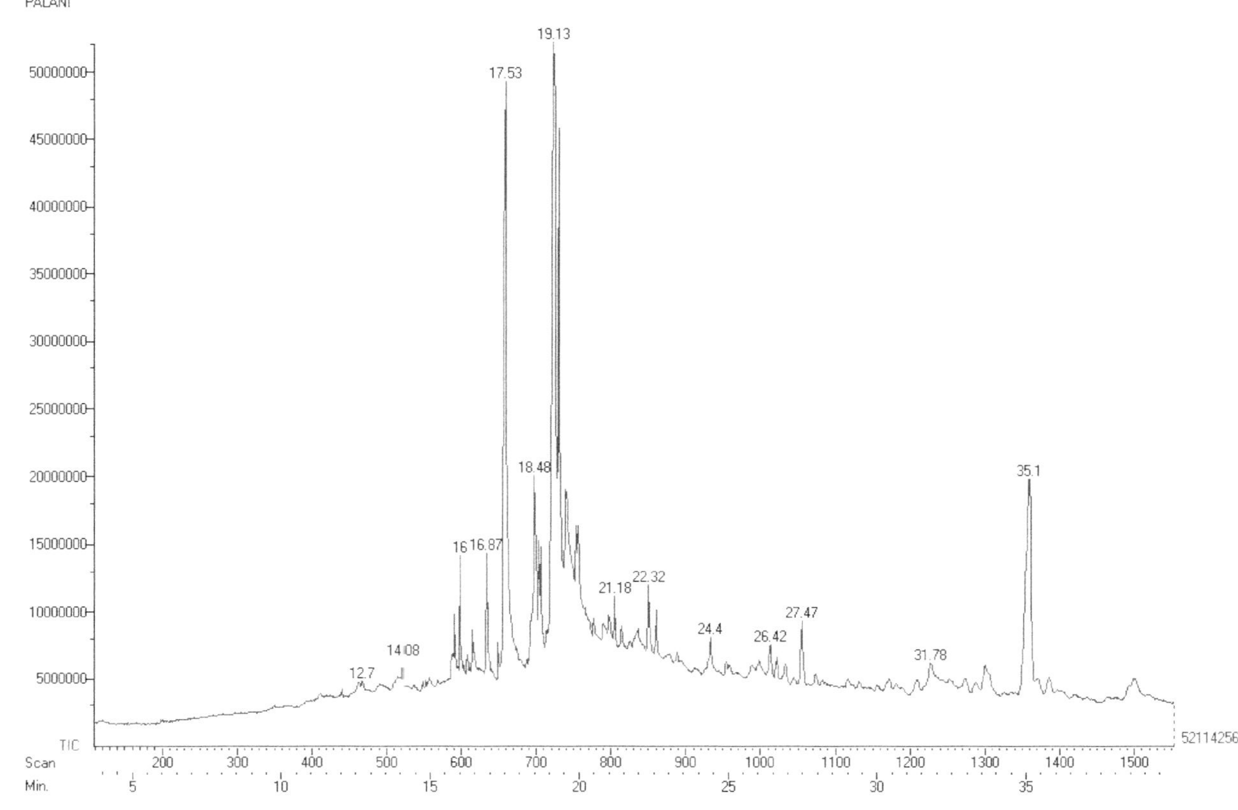

Figure 26: GC/MS analysis of methanolic crude extract of *C. albidum*

RT	Chemical name	Chemical formula	Molecular weight (g/mol)
12.7	1-isopropyl-4-methylcyclohexa-1,4-diene	$C_{10}H_{16}$	136.23
14.08	Phenol, 2,4-bis-(1,1-dimethylethyl)	C17H30OSi	278.511
16	Flavone	C15H10O2	222.24
16.87	6-methoxy flavone	C16H12O3	252.26
17.53	palmitic acid	C16H32O2	256.42
18.7	oleic acid	C18H34O2	282.46
19.13	Phytol	C20H40O	296.53
21.18	Coumarine, 3-[2-(1-methyl-2-imidazolylthio)-1-oxoethyl]-	C15H12N2O3S	300.33238
22.32	4-(benzyloxy)-4-(2,2-dimethyl-1,3-dioxolan-4-yl)butanal	$C_{16}H_{22}O_4$	278.34
24.4	Stigmasterol	C29H48O	412.702
26.42	Corynan-17-ol, 18,19-didehydro-10-methoxy-, acetate (ester)	C22H28N2O3	368.477
	Pregna-4,6-diene-3,20-dione, 17-(acetyloxy)-6-methyl-	C24H32O4	384.516
31.78	Azafrin	C27H38O4	426.597
35.1	6-Bromo-1,1,4,4,7-pentamethyl-1,2,3,4-tetrahydronaphthalene	C15H21Br	281.237

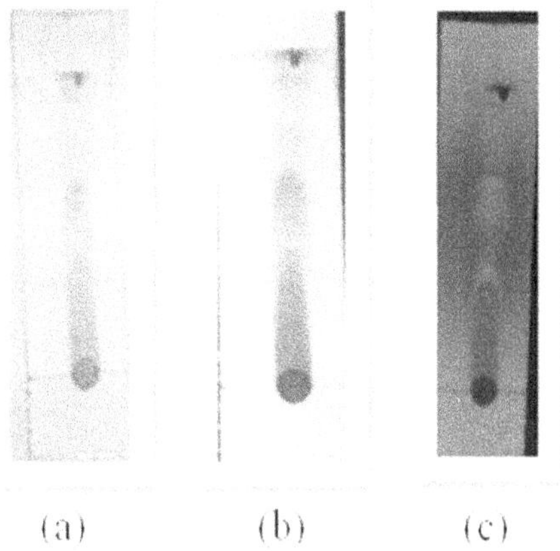

(a)   (b)   (c)

Figure 27. Thin layer chromatography of *C. albidum* methanol extract (a) visible light, (b) short UV, (c) long UV

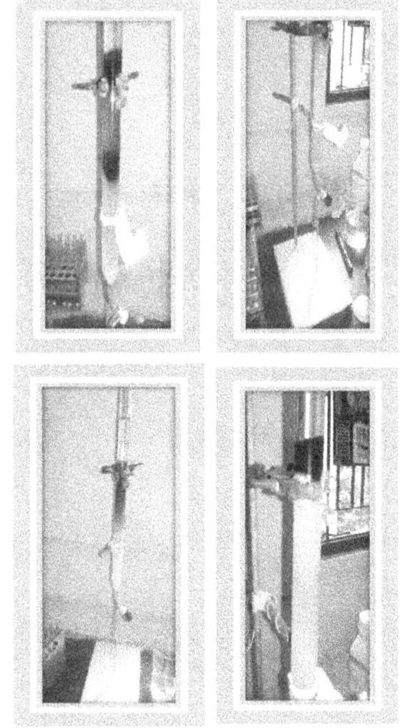

Figure 28. Column chromatography setup for separation of *C. albidum* methanol extract

4.9 CHARACTERIZATION OF ACTIVE FRACTION CA1

4.9.1 ULTRAVIOLET (UV) VISIBLE SPECTRUM OF CA1 FRACTION

For the UV spectrum of the CA1 compound, the highest peak was observed at 257 nm (**Figure 29**). In General, isoflavones are detected in the UV wavelength of 250- 265 nm.

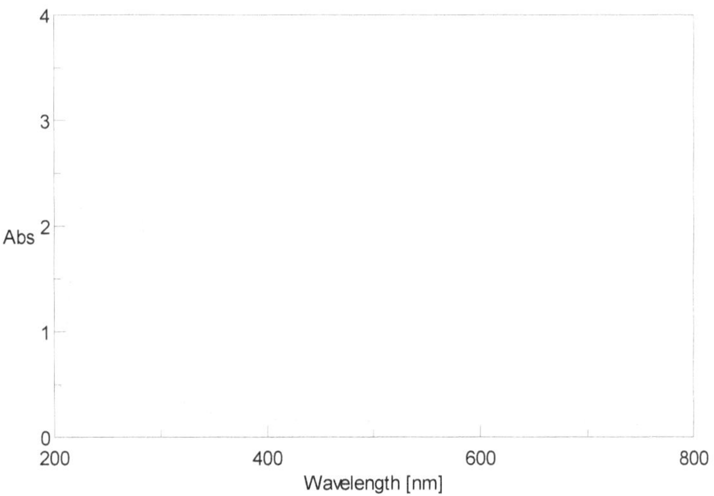

Figure 29: Ultraviolet (UV) Visible Spectrum of Fraction CA1

4.9.2 FOURIER TRANSFORM- INFRA-RED (FTIR) SPECTRUM OF CA1 FRACTION

The FTIR spectrum is used to identify the functional group of the isolated fraction CA1. The spectrum reveals that the peak value of 3065 cm-1 corresponds to (OH) hydroxyl group, 1675 cm-1 and 1596 cm-1 represents the presence of (C=O) carbonyl group. The bands at 1446 cm-1 and 1506 cm-1 exhibits the C=C group. The methyl group (-CH3) arising in the regions of 1240 cm-1, 1177 cm-1, 1080 cm-1 and 1014 cm-1, respectively (**Figure 30**).

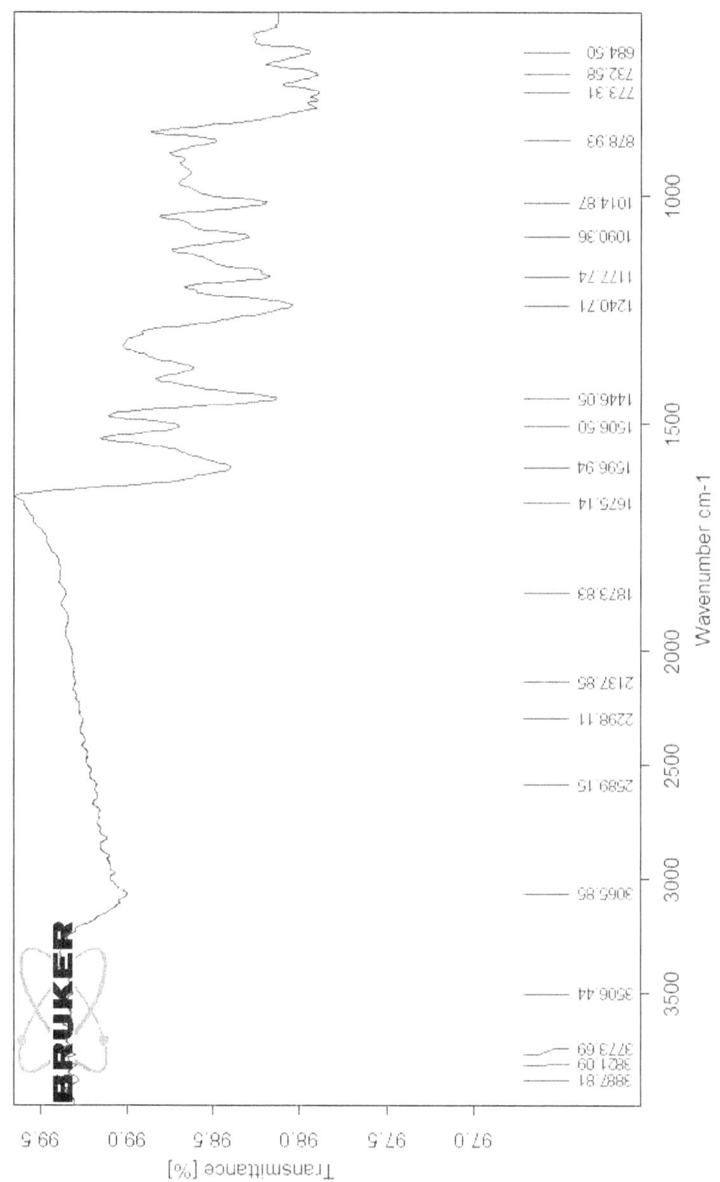

Figure 30. : FTIR spectrum of CA1 compound

4.9.3 NUCLEAR MAGNETIC RESONANCE (NMR) SPECTRUM OF CA1 FRACTION

The NMR spectrum was used to elucidate the structure of isolated compound CA1. ^{13}C NMR spectrum facilitates to find out the position and number of carbon atoms present in the molecule. The ^{13}C NMR spectrum results totally of 16 carbon atoms. The signal at δ 55.5 corresponds to OMe, the C-2 presents at δ 153.6 followed by C-3 at δ124.7, C-4 at δ 175.07, C-5 at 127.7 regions (**Figure 31**). The signal at δ 115.6 corresponds to C-6, δ 163.02 for C-7 and δ102.5 represents C-8 position. The C-9 was present in the region of δ 157.9 and C-10 was present δ 117.9. The C-11 to C-16 was presented in the regions of δ123.6, δ130.5, δ 114.05 and δ 159.4, respectively.

The ^{1}H NMR spectrums are used to determine the position and amount of protons present in the molecule. There are totally 12 hydrogen atoms were recorded in the ^{1}H NMR spectrum (**Figure 32**). The peak rising from δ3.78 corresponds to 3H- OCH3, followed by a peak at δ 6.87 represents H-8 and the peak at δ 6.95 was H-6. The signal at δ6.97 contains two protons at a place of H-3' and H-5', likewise the signal at δ7.51 also contains two protons which are H-2'and H- 6'. The signals at δ 7.96 and δ 8.33 are leads to H- 2and H- 5. The peak at δ 10.80 corresponds to the OH group, respectively.

4.9.4 GAS CHROMATOGRAPHY AND MASS SPECTRUM (GC/MS) OF CA1 FRACTION

Gas chromatography and Mass spectrum (GC/MS) is used to identify and to check the purity of the compound CA1. The gas chromatogram results in the presence of a single peak in the retention time of 4.19 with an area of 100% (**Figure 33**). In the meantime, the mass spectrum of compound CA1 illustrates the spectral value of 267.36 m/z (**Figure 34**).

Based on the spectral characterization the isolated CA1 was corresponding to 7-Hydroxy-4'-methoxy isoflavone (formononetin). The molecular formula of obtained compound 7-Hydroxy-4'-methoxy isoflavone was $C_{16}H_{12}O_4$ and the molecular weight was 268.29 g/ mol^{-1}. The melting point of the compound was 256-258°C.

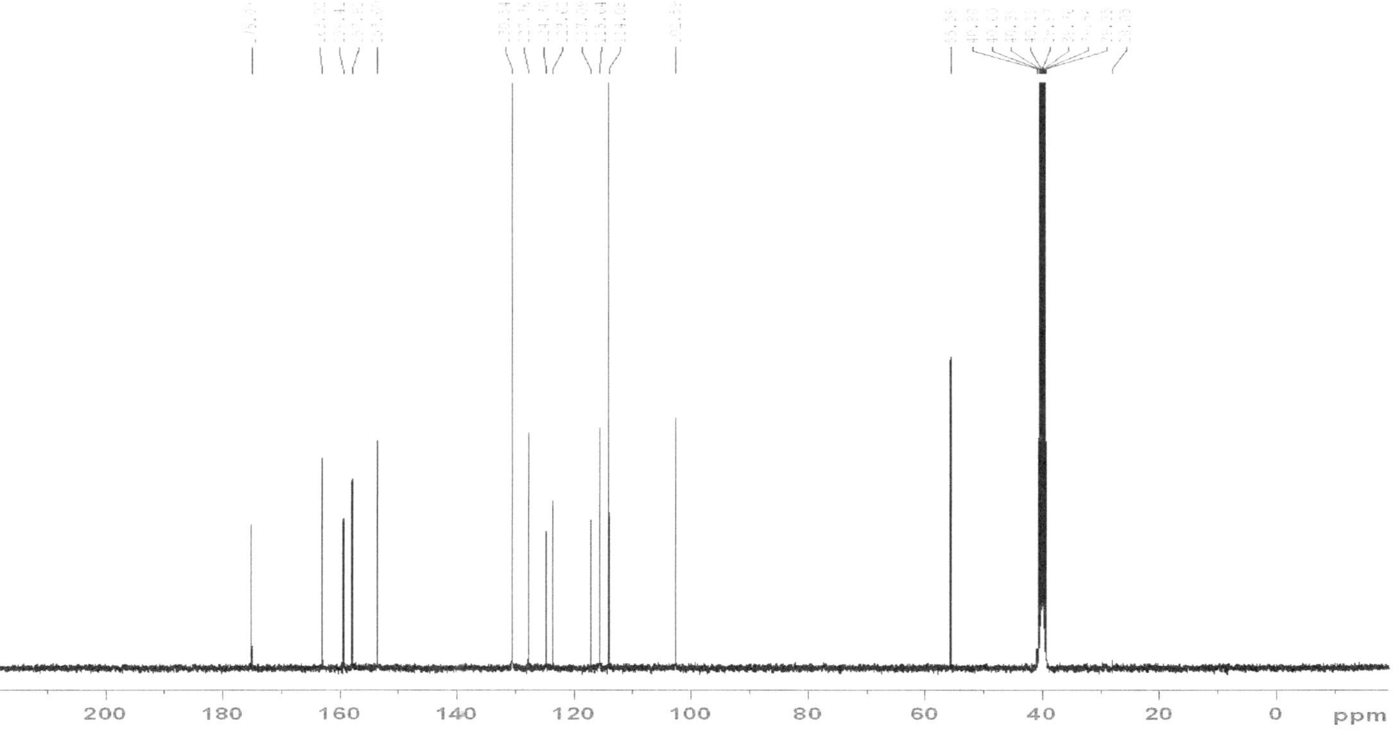

Figure 31. ^{13}C NMR spectrum of CA1 compound

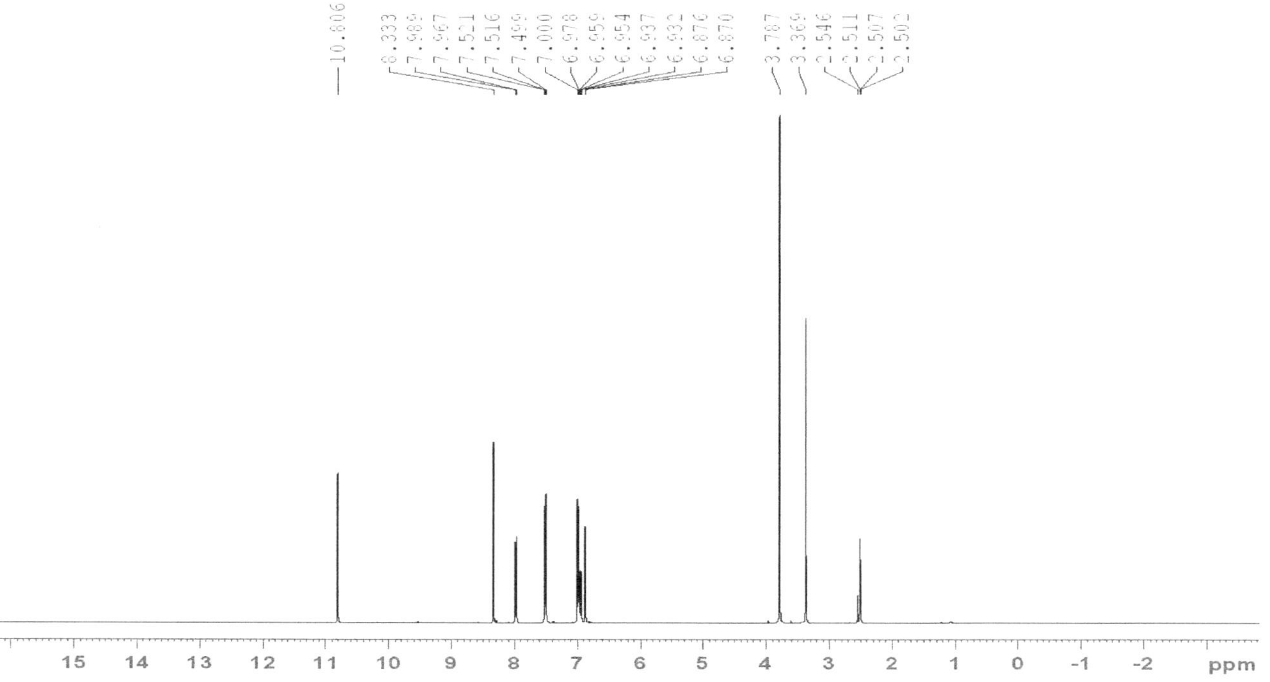

Figure 32. ^{1}H NMR spectrum of CA1 compound

Figure 33. Gas Chromatogram of CA1 compound

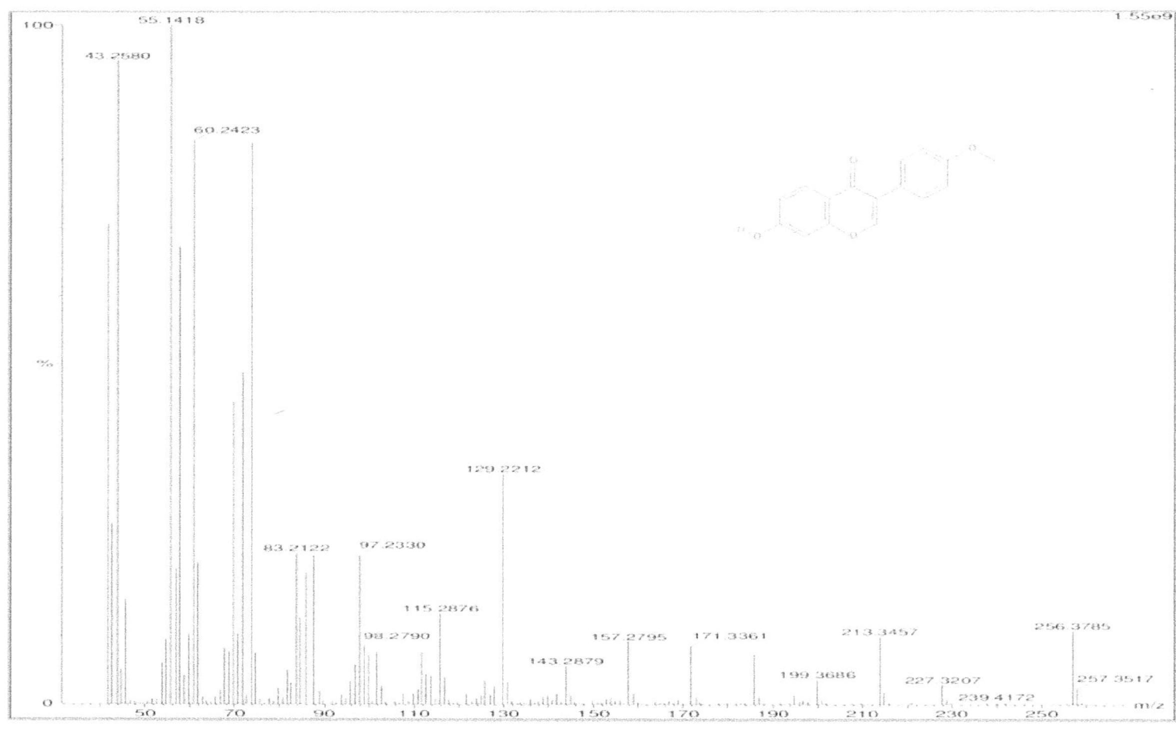

Figure 34. Mass Spectrum of CA1 compound

4.10 DETERMINATION OF ANTIOXIDANT ACTIVITY OF 7-HYDROXY-4'-METHOXYISOFLAVONE

4.10.1 (DPPH) 2,2-DIPHENYLPICRYLHYDRAZYL RADICAL SCAVENGING ACTIVITY OF CA1 COMPOUND

The DPPH radical scavenging activity was measured by a reduction in the absorbance value at 517 nm. The DPPH radical scavenging ability of CA1 exhibited significant effect in a dose-dependent manner (5- 25 µg/ml) in the reaction mixture. The inhibition percentage of CA1 was 87.13% with an IC_{50} value of 13.05 µg/ml and ascorbic acid was 91.23% with an IC_{50} value of 8.60 µg/ml (**Figure 35**). The results revealed that the DPPH radical scavenging capacity of CA1 is comparable to ascorbic acid, which indicates the nearly potency of compound.

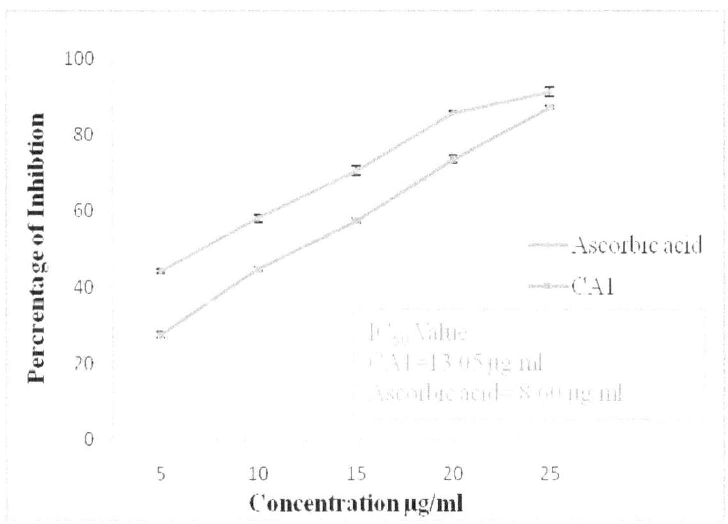

Figure 35. DPPH radical Scavenging assay of compound CA1

4.10.2 HYDROXYL (*OH) RADICAL SCAVENGING ACTIVITY OF CA1 COMPOUND

The hydroxyl radical scavenging ability of CA1 was determined by different concentrations as 25, 50, 75, 100, 125 and 150 µg/ml. The result shows the inhibition percentage of 12.98, 28.68, 34.42, 41.86, 48.76 and 53.19% with fifty percentage inhibition concentration of 141 µg/ml, respectively. The inhibition percentage of ascorbic acid was 67.75% and fifty percentage inhibition concentration was113.73 µg/ml. The results clearly explained that the inhibition percentage of CA1 near to ascorbic which acid was in a dose-dependent manner (**Figure 36**).

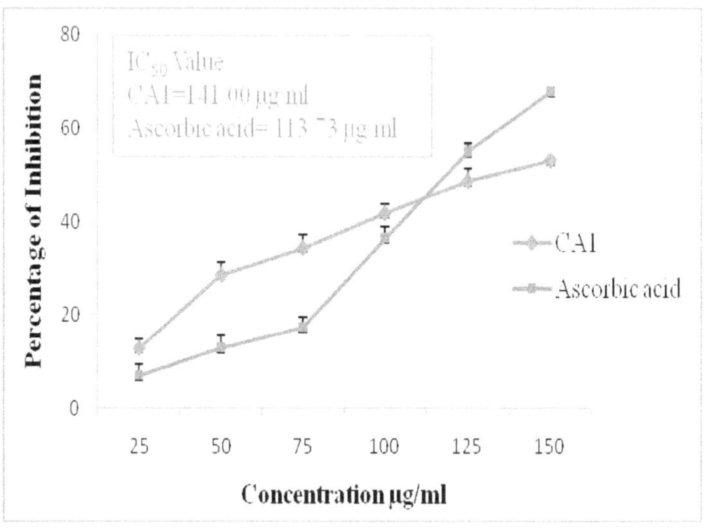

Figure 36. Hydroxyl radical Scavenging assay of compound CA1

4.10.3 SUPEROXIDE ANION (O$_2^-$) RADICAL SCAVENGING ACTIVITY CA1 COMPOUND

The superoxide radical scavenging activity of CA1 was determined by the nitro blue tetrazolium method. The reduction of absorbance value at 560 nm points out the compound or mixture utilizes the superoxide anion. The result of CA1 and standard ascorbic acid shows 89.25% and   95.33% at 30 µg/ml, respectively (**Figure 37**). The IC$_{50}$ values of CA1 and ascorbic acid was 13.05 µg/ml and 9.46 µg/ml. However, the superoxide scavenging ability of CA1 was low when compared to ascorbic acid, but significant.

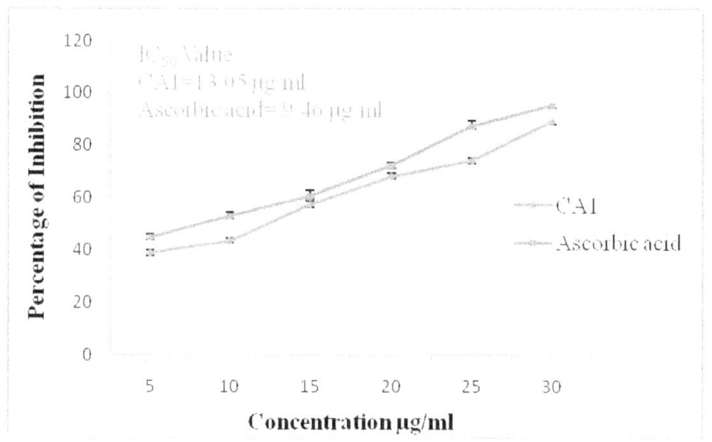

Figure 37. Super oxide radical Scavenging assay of compound CA1

4.10.4 NITRIC OXIDE (NO) RADICAL SCAVENGING ACTIVITY OF CA1 COMPOUND

The CA1 shows strong nitric oxide radical scavenging activity of 49.78, 65.25, 70.95, 81.07, 83.63 and 85.74% at various concentrations as 20, 40, 60, 80, 100 and 120 µg/ml, respectively (**Figure 38**). The inhibition percentage of ascorbic acid was 93.28% at a higher concentration of 120 µg/ml. The IC_{50} value of CA1 was 30.65 µg/ml, whereas ascorbic acid was 16.44 µg/ml, respectively.

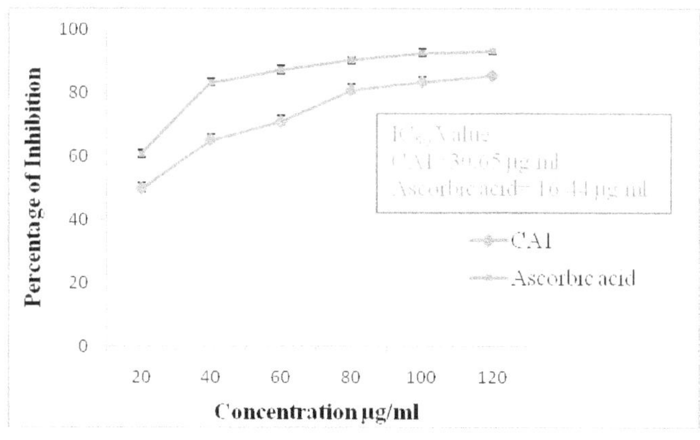

Figure 38. Nitric oxide radical Scavenging assay of compound CA1

4.11 ANTIINFLAMMATORY ACTIVITY

4.11.1 EFFECTS OF CRUDE EXTRACT AND ON THE VIABILITY OF RAW 264.7 MACROPHAGES

The effects of the crude extract and fraction on the viability of RAW 264.7 cells *in vitro* by incubating cells with different concentrations (5-320µg/ml) studied and the results of MTT assay demonstrated no cytotoxicity to RAW macrophages even at concentrations up to 320µg/ml (**Figure 39 and Figure 40**).

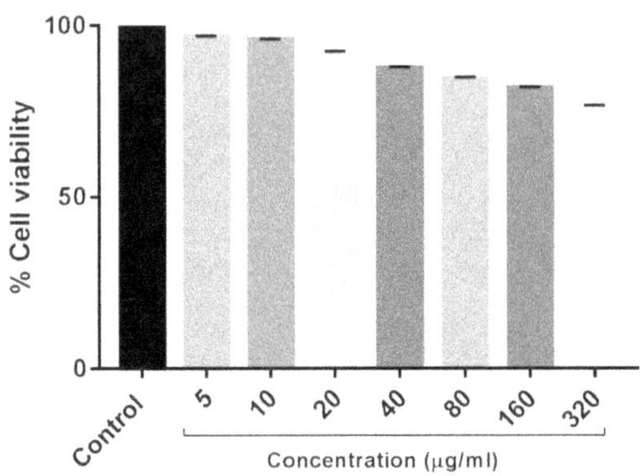

Figure 39. Effect of crude extract on the viability of RAW 264.7 macrophages

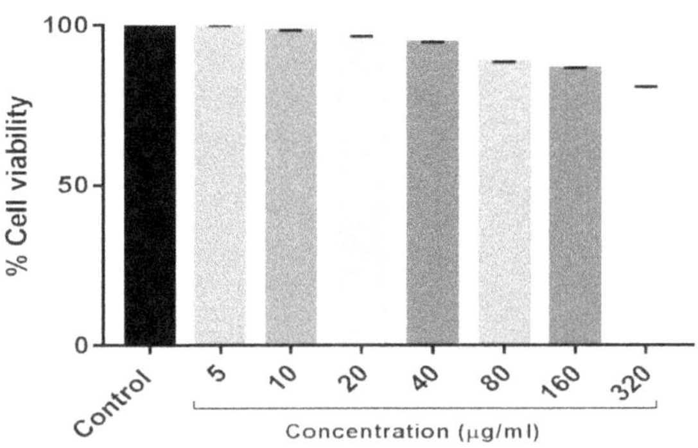

Figure 40. Effect of CA1 on the viability of RAW 264.7 macrophages

4.11.2 EFFECTS OF CA1 ON LPS-INDUCED NO PRODUCTION AND iNOS EXPRESSION

The anti-inflammatory activity of the CA1 fraction was investigated on LPS-stimulated RAW 264.7 mouse macrophages. Macrophages, on activation with toxins such as lipopolysaccharides (LPS), initiate a cascade of inflammatory events that are mediated by a wide range of markers. LPS-stimulated macrophages produce inflammatory mediators such as free radicals, NO, iNOS and IL-6. The effect of the plant fraction on LPS-induced NO production and inducible nitric oxide synthase (iNOS) was determined by incubating the macrophages in different concentrations of the fraction. After 24h of incubation, the nitrate levels in the supernatants were found to be significantly ($p<0.001$) decreased when compared to the LPS alone treated group. The inhibition was found to be declined by up to 22% at 320µg/ml. The IC_{50} value was calculated and was found to be 55.57µg/ml. Hence, further gene expression studies were carried out using 27.5, 55 and 110µg/ml concentrations. The results of the effect of CA1 on LPS induced NO production and iNOS expression were showed in **Figure 41 and Figure 42**. The gene expression of iNOS, the enzyme which synthesizes NO was also evaluated. It was observed from the results that LPS alone has upregulated the iNOS level which was significantly ($p<0.001$) down-regulated in the plant fraction treated groups.

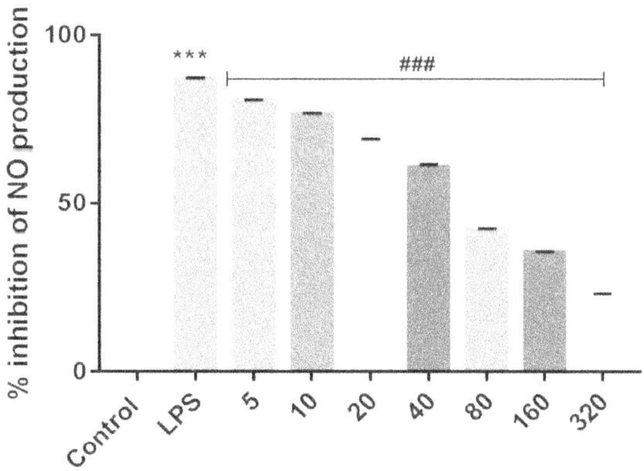

Figure 41. Effect of CA1 on LPS-induced NO production

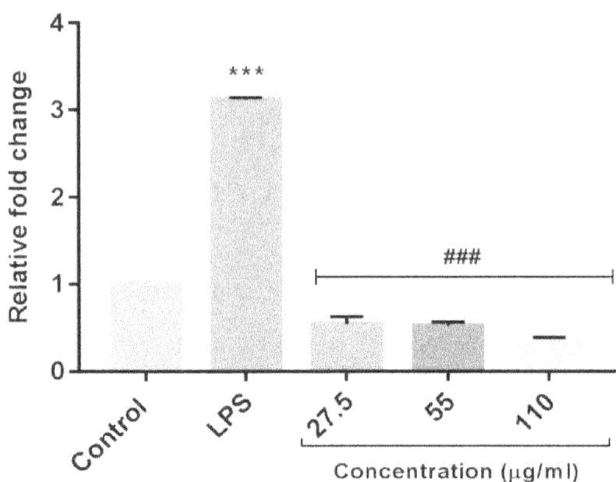

Figure 42. Effect of CA1 on LPS-induced iNOS expression

4.11.3 EFFECT OF COMPOUND CA1 ON PRO- INFLAMMATORY AND ANTI-INFLAMMATORY CYTOKINES

In order to further evaluate the anti-inflammatory mechanism in detail, the expression of key pro- and anti-inflammatory cytokines was evaluated by quantitative real-time PCR. The effect of plant fractions on the production of the pro-inflammatory cytokines TNF-α, IL-1β and IL-6, and the anti-inflammatory cytokine IL-10 was measured in the culture medium of macrophages stimulated with 1µg/ml of LPS alone or in combination with different concentrations of the plant fraction. The expression of COX-2 was also evaluated. The results of the present study showed that LPS stimulated the expression of pro-inflammatory cytokines IL- 1β, IL-6 and TNF-α (**Figure 43, 44 & Figure 45**). COX-2 was also found to be upregulated in the LPS-induced group (**Figure 46**), whereas the gene expression of anti-inflammatory cytokine IL-10 was found down-regulated (**Figure 47**).

The plant fraction at the tested concentrations of 27.5, 55 and 110µg/ml has significantly down-regulated the expression of pro-inflammatory cytokines and the COX-2 expression. The anti-inflammatory cytokine IL-10 showed increased expression when compared to LPS-alone induced group.

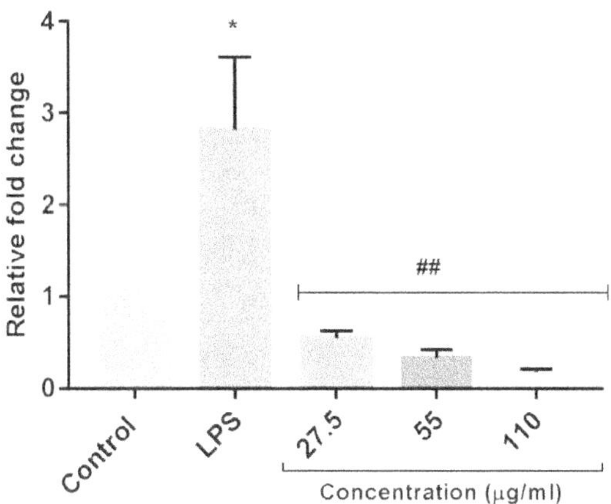

Figure 43. Effect of CA1 on pro- inflammatory cytokines 1L-1β

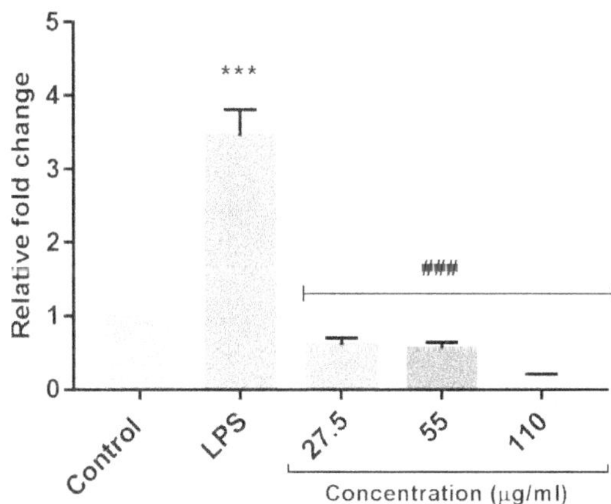

Figure 44. Effect of CA1 on pro- inflammatory cytokines 1L-6

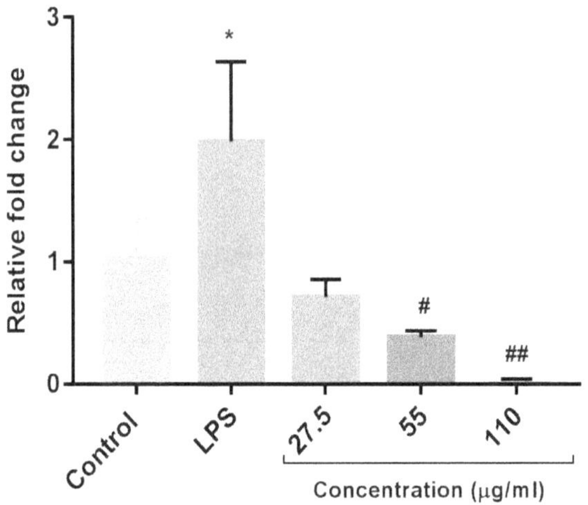

Figure 45. Effect of CA1 on pro- inflammatory cytokines TNF-α

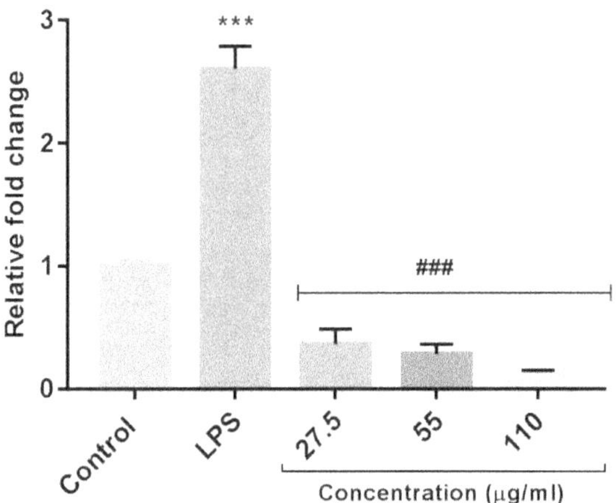

Figure 46. Effect of CA1 on COX-2 expression

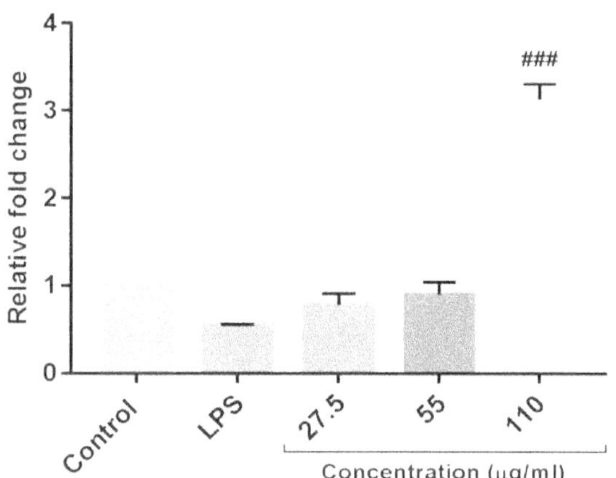

Figure 47. Effect of CA1 on anti-inflammatory cytokines 1L-10

4.12 ANTICANCER ACTIVITY OF COMPOUND CA1 AND PLANT CRUDE EXTRACT ON HELA HUMAN CERVICAL CANCER CELL LINES

4.12.1 CYTOTOXICITY ASSAY

The *in vitro* anticancer activity of CA1 and crude extract on HeLa human cervical cancer cell line were examined by using MTT assay. The HeLa human cervical cancer cells were treated with CA1 and crude extract in different concentrations as 5, 10, 20, 40, 80, 160 and 320 µg/ml. The inhibition percentage of CA1 was 78.32 %, whereas crude extract consists of 61.38% at higher concentrations of 320 µg/ml. The fifty percentage inhibition concentration of CA1 was 108.25 µg/ml, while 260.67 µg/ml for methanolic crude extract, respectively **(Figure 48 and Figure 49)**. The treatment of methanolic crude extract and CA1 against HeLa human cervical cancer cells on the treatment of different concentrations and their morphological changes were presented in **(Figure 50 & 51)**. The results clearly indicate that HeLa human cervical cancer cells were effectively inhibited by CA1 when compared to methanolic extract.

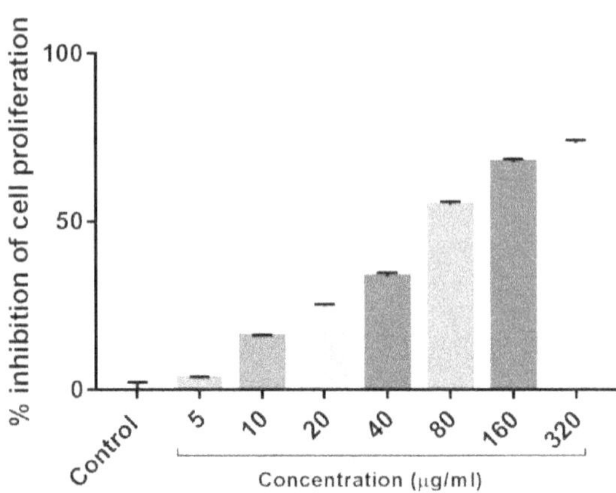

Figure 48. Effect of *C. albidum* crude extract on HeLa human cervical cancer cell line by using MTT assay

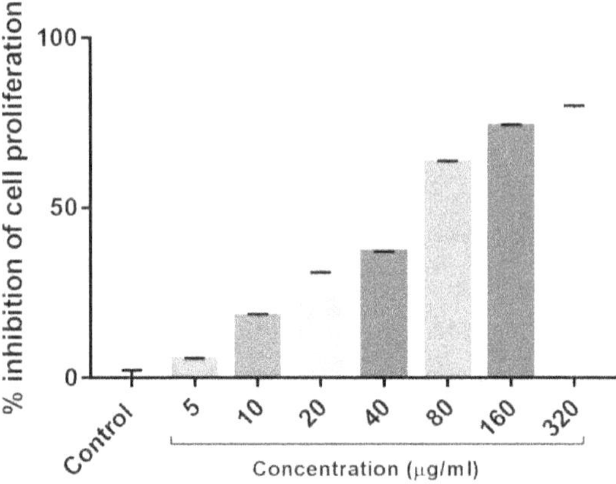

Figure 49. Effect of CA1 on HeLa human cervical cancer cell line by using MTT assay

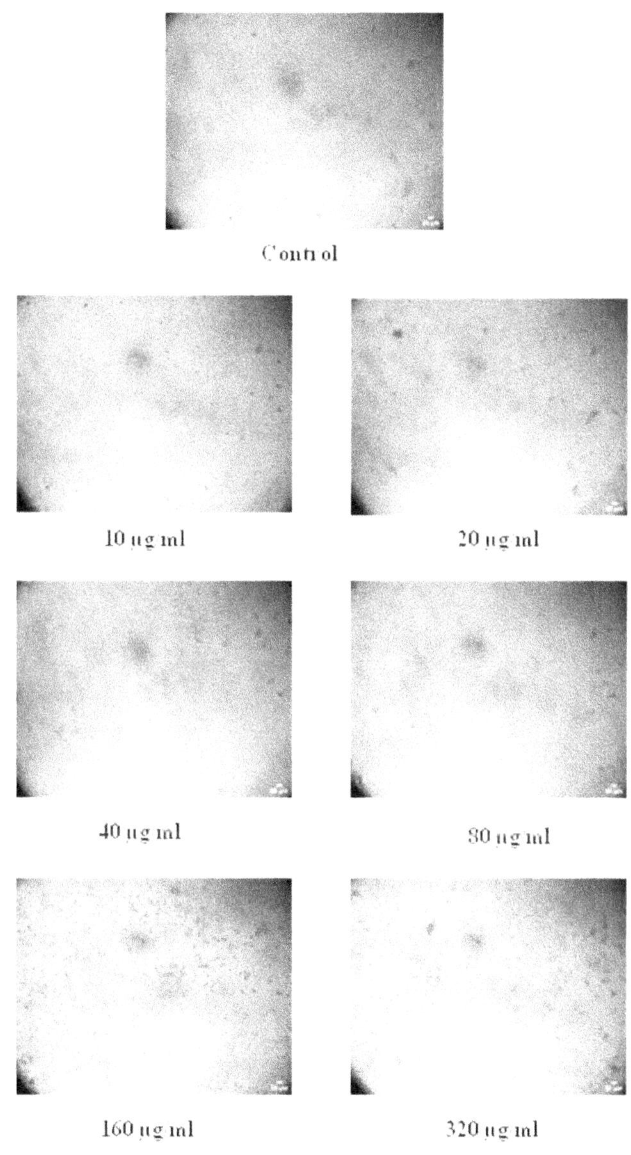

Figure 50. Photomicrograph of morphological changes observed in HeLa cervical cancer cells on different concentrations *C. albidum* methanolic extract following 24h incubation (10x magnification)

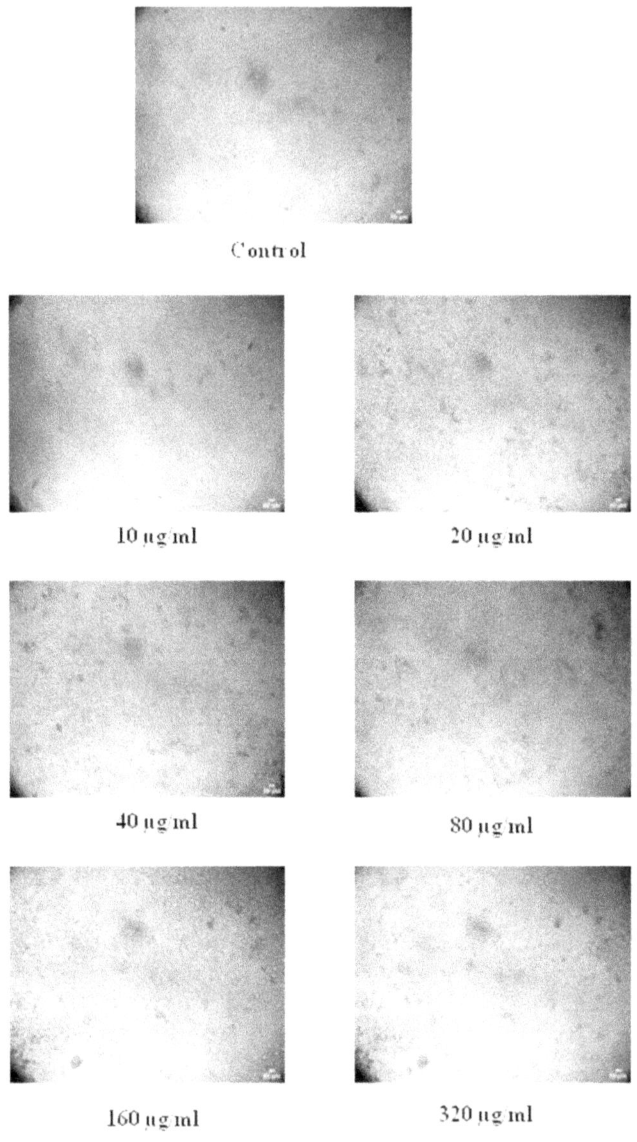

Figure 51. Photomicrograph of morphological changes observed in HeLa cervical cancer cells on different concentrations CA1 following 24h incubation (10x magnification)

4.12.2 ETHIDIUM BROMIDE/ACRIDINE ORANGE STAIINNG (DUAL STAINING)

The treated and untreated HeLa cells were labelled with Acridine Orange/ Ethidium Bromide stain. The fluorescent microscope was used to determine the induction of apoptosis based on the appearance of the stained color on HeLa cells. The green fluorescence indicates the presence of live cells or untreated cells. The treatment of stained cells was based on IC_{50} concentrations of CA1. The early-stage apoptotic cells were identified by the presence of yellow colour fluorescence and the orange stained cells indicate the presence of late-stage apoptotic cells. The dead cells or necrotic cells were notified by the presence of red color cells (**Figure 52**). Based on the above observations, it is observed that the CA1 increases the apoptosis induction on higher concentrations and length of the treatment period. The CA1 induces apoptosis at 39.43% at a lower concentration of 54 µg/ml and 80.61% at a higher concentration of 108 µg/ml (**Figure 53**).

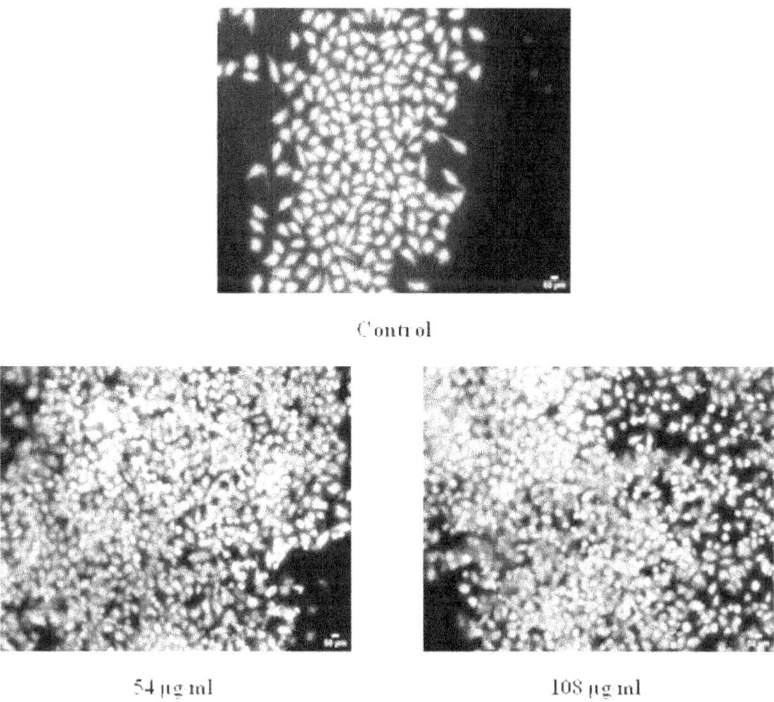

Figure 52. Morphological changes observed in HeLa cells on CA1 by EB/AO staining assay

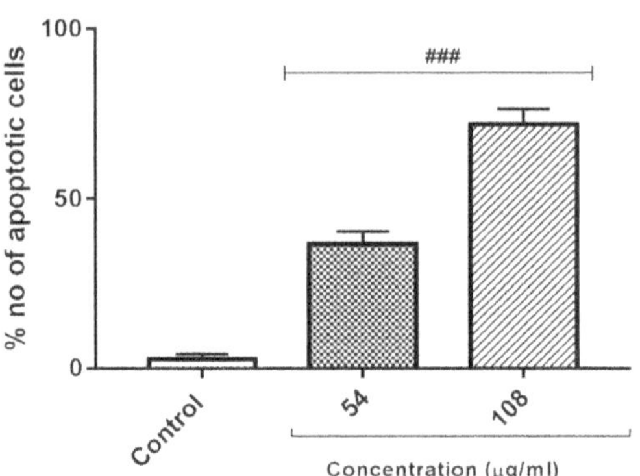

Figure 53. The effect of CA1 on the induction of apoptosis in HeLa9 cells

4.12.3 REACTIVE OXYGEN SPECIES TEST (ROS)

The 2′,7′-Dichlorofluorescein staining was widely used to evaluate the intracellular reactive oxygen species (ROS) generation. The stimulation of ROS generation was measured by the increasing green fluorescent intensity which indicates the apoptotic stimulation. The treatment of CA1on ROS generation results in an increase of fluorescence intensity in a dose-dependent manner. The microscopic images of CA1 treated cells were clearly given away that the development of green fluorescence in cells was due to an increase in concentration **(Figure 54)**. Fluorescence intensity of lower dose (54 µg/ml) treated cells shows 46.43% and higher dose (108 µg/ml) contains 75.61%, respectively **(Figure 55)**.

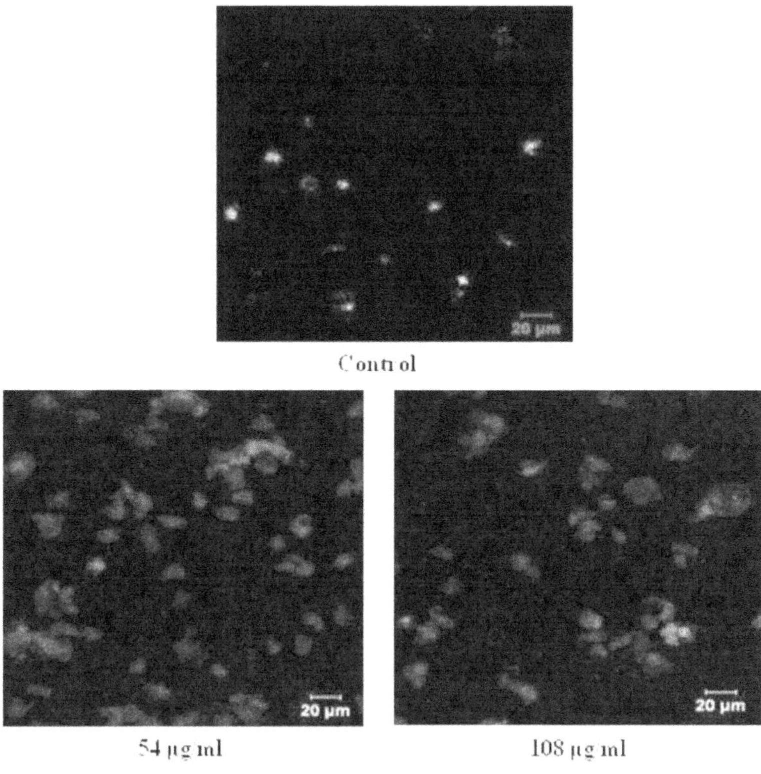

Figure 54. Microscopic images showing enhanced green fluorescence confirms ROS inhibition (10x Magnification)

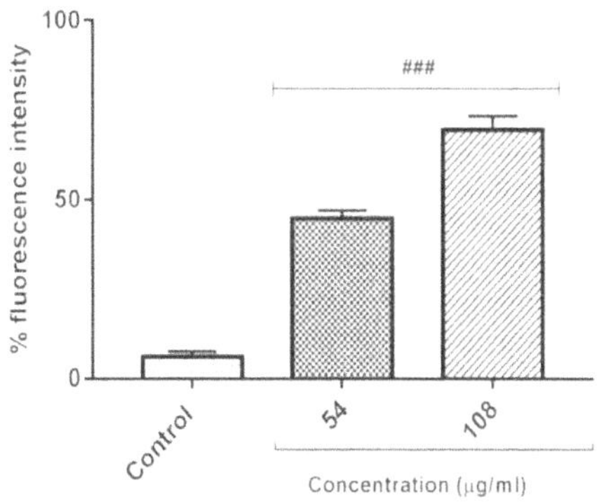

Figure 55. The effect of CA1 on the inhibition of ROS in HeLa9 cells

4.12.4 FLOWCYTOMETRY ANALYSIS

The flow cytometry analysis was used to determine the range of cell cycle checkpoints. Propidium Iodide (PI) is broadly used for cell viability techniques. The dye was prohibited by apoptotic cells due to the preserved cytoplasm membrane, whereas necrotic cells accept the dye attribute to the damaged cell membrane and induce red fluorescence. Flow cytometry analysis was used to examine the effect of CA1on HeLa cervical cancer cell cycle distribution in different phases. The results explained that cells exposed to a significant increase in the accumulation of the DNA contents in the G0/G1 phase (**Figure 56**). Both S and G2/M phase cells decreased in the treatment. It has been observed that CA1 arresting cells in the G0/G1 phase of the cell cycle.

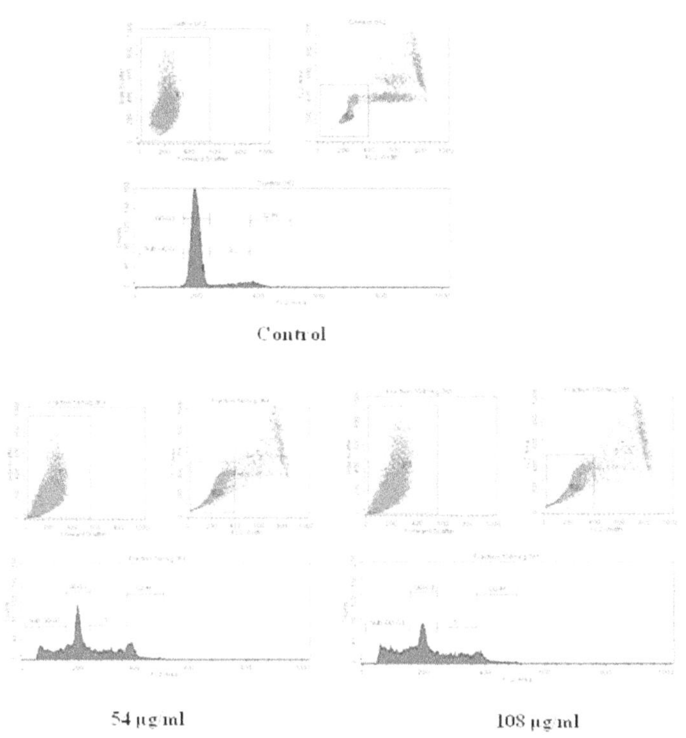

Figure 56. : Effect of CA1 on the redistribution of cells in different phases of cell cycle

4.12.5 GENE EXPRESSION ANALYSIS RT-PCR ANALYSIS

The study was intended to examine CA1 induced apoptosis through the promising signalling pathways. RT-PCR technique is used to analysis of the gene expression of anti-apoptotic and pro-apoptotic genes like Bcl-2, Bax, caspase-3, caspase-9 and cytochrome c in HeLa cervical cancer cells. As mentioned in the (**Figure 57**), anti-apoptotic protein Bcl-2 level was decreased, meanwhile, the pro-apoptotic proteins like Bax, caspase-3, caspase-9, and cytochrome c were increased in low dose and high dose (**Figure 58 to Figure 61**). Based on the study, the result strongly reveals that CA1 enhancement of the pro-apoptotic genes and down-regulates the anti-apoptotic gene resulted to increase the apoptosis.

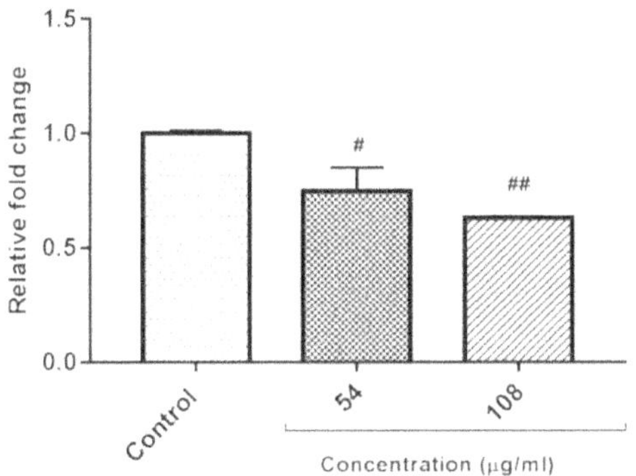

Figure 57. Relative Fold change in Bcl-2 gene expression between the control and treatment

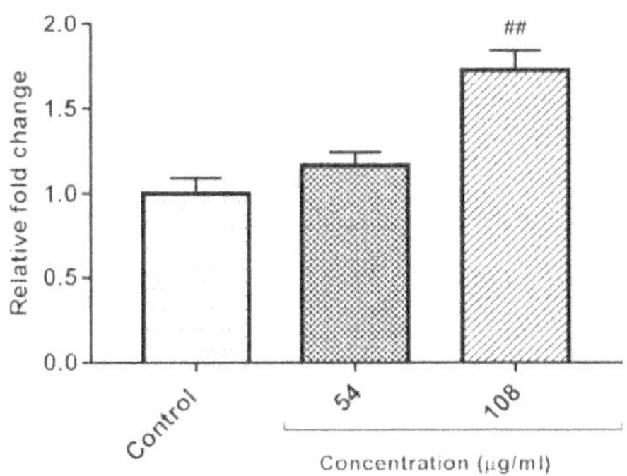

Figure 58. Relative Fold change in Bax gene expression between the control and treatment

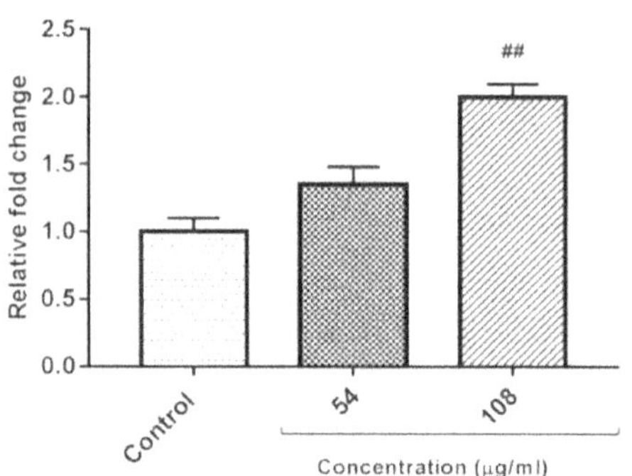

Figure 59. Relative Fold change in Caspase 3 gene expression between the control and treatment

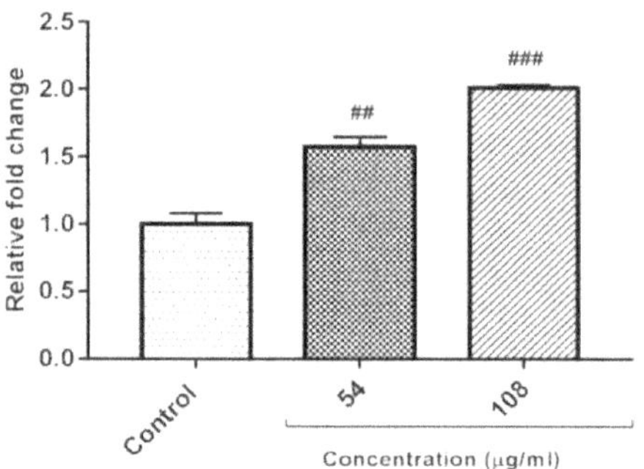

Figure 60. Relative Fold change in Caspase 9 gene expression between the control and treatment

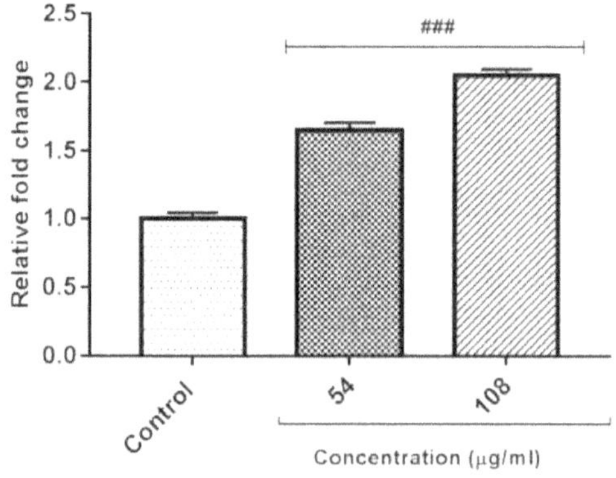

Figure 61. Relative Fold change in cytochrome c expression between the control and treatment

DISCUSSION

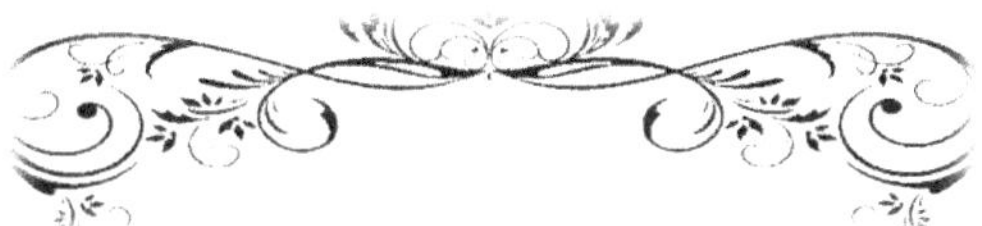

CHAPTER- V

DISCUSSION

In the current scenario, herbal medicines are considered as the oldest type of health care system. In the earliest period of improvement in development of new medicine, traditional medicine systems progress more than centuries by different communities. They have still maintained an enormous knowledge of traditional medicines (Mukherjee and Wahil, 2006). The knowledge, practice and skills were used in traditional folk medicine with supporting beliefs, theories and understanding it's indigenous for maintenance of health. Whereas an ethnobotanical survey plays a major role in the conservation and utilization of biological resources by proper documentation. The ethnobotanical survey is the most important and consistent way of making drug discovery (Kolanjinathan and Saranraj, 2015;

Saranraj *et al.*, 2016). Hence, the ethnobotanical investigation was carried out in Thiruvadisoolam village, Kancheepuram District of Tamil Nadu, India in the present study to find out method of use of traditional medicine. The survey study reports 54 species of medicinal plants belonging to 46 Genera and 35 families which are used for various ailments, which corroborates the earlier reports of Muthu *et al.* (2006) and Selvadurai *et al.* (2018) on ethnobotanical survey of Kanchipuram area and that support the observations of present study.

Indian traditional medicine systems mainly depend on medicinal plants which frequently used plant parts such as leaves and roots (Giday *et al.*, 2003; Wondimu *et al.*, 2007). The present investigation revealed that most of the common disease of human are cured by plants, where the herbal healers used many plant parts such as leaves and plants used most frequently, followed by seeds and aerial parts respectively. The study area Thiruvadisoolam is little distant from the town, hence the local people are mainly depending on the plants for the first aids in emergency situations like snack bite, scorpion bite, insect bites, stomach disorders, cut injuries and various allergic diseases. Since, most of the elders are not showing interest to avail the allopathic medicine for their illness, the herbal healers treats those patient in this system of medicine. From the survey, it was observed that as the treatment procedures are not opened one, the healers are maintaining secrecy with the public, but they thought their family member who are showing real interest will be discussed the herbal medicinal system.

The healers treating even much serious illness with the uses of plants, but they are not aware of the phytocompounds present in the plants. Based on the literature survey, the study area contains very few reports on the information of phytochemistry of plants present. However, there is no remarkable scientific-based surveys are reported in the study area. The plant diversity is varying in different seasons of the year, more plants are seen in the rainy seasons and less population in summer. Hence, the study area was selected for ethnobotanical survey based on the richness in vegetation and its usage information from uses on face to face interview method. In the neighbouring geographical regions, the people are not showing interest in the plant based ailments due to various reasons such as the similar studies on medicinal plants and it utilization in healthcare are found which are comparable with their conservation and utilization that has been carried out in various places of India (Ayyanar and Ignacimuthu, 2011; Xavier *et al.*, 2014; Shil *et al.*, 2014; Xavier *et al.*, 2015).

The earlier reports of ethnobotanical study in Kancheepuram district of Tamil Nadu shows the traditional healers used 9 species of medicinal plants for stomach pain and digestive problems (Muthu *et al.*, 2006). The frequent use of leaves than other parts of plants which are used by the traditional healers in the present study was in agreement with the previous reports that the herbal medicine was prepared most frequently with plant leaves around the world (Ghorbani, 2005; Ullah *et al.*, 2013; Morvin Yabesh *et al.*, 2014; Vijayakumar *et al.*, 2015). Moreover, the plant leaves are uncomplicated to collect rather than other plant parts such as flowers, seeds and fruits which are available mostly in particular season, whereas barks are plant damaged surface tissues. In addition, the leaves are actively functioned through photosynthesis and produce primary and secondary metabolites which are involved in bioactive constituents of plants (Amri and Kisangau, 2012). The stem bark of *Combretum albidum* was used for the treatment of jaundice by Chinnar tribal people from the Idukki District of Kerala (Sreedhar *et al.*, 2012), which is in resemblance with the present ethnobotanical observation.

Based on the documentation of the ethnomedicinal studies and usage by the healers, 10 plants selected in the present study such as *Z. Officinale, S. nux-vomica, G. asiatica, E. hirta, P. emblica, C. auriculata, C. retusa, C. spinarum, C. albidum* and *K. reticulata* to assess various biological activities. The results of the preliminary screening of qualitative phytochemical analysis of the 10 selected plants revealed the presence of alkaloids, phenols, glycosides, terpenoids, flavonoids, tannins, reducing sugars, saponins, proteins and steroids the quantity ranging from lower level to higher level might be the reasons for medicinal properties which is in coincidence with the previous findings as the secondary metabolites reported to have effective biological and therapeutic properties (Narender *et al.*, 2012; Vishnu *et al.*, 2013; Benedec *et al.*, 2013; Charalampos *et al.*, 2013).

According to Sreedhar *et al.* (2012), the methanolic extract of *C. albidum* stem bark contains flavonoids, tannins, triterpenes, glycosides and saponins the similar phytochemicals were reported in the present investigation, which coincidence to the present study. Flavonoids, tannins and triterpenoids are major phytoconstituents which found to acts as hepatoprotection agents was reported by several authors Absar *et al.*, (2007); Manjunatha and Vidya, (2008); Das and Sarma, (2009). Alkaloids and saponins were reported to present in leaves, stem, flower, and fruit of *C. albidum* G. Don which is used for the treatments of heart-related diseases, diarrhea, dysentery and inflammation (Bokhad and Rothe, 2012). Many researchers reported that *Combretum* spp. contain flavonoids, anthracene glycosides, coumarins, steroids, tannins, triterpenoids and saponins, Raveesha (2015) which witnessed for the findings of *C. albidum* in the present study.

The different solvents and extraction methods are reliable for isolating endogenous compounds from different parts of the plant materials (Siddhuraju and Becker, 2003). Phenolics are abundantly present in plant material which is predominantly used in the food industry due to antioxidant property through oxidative degradation of lipids, increase nutritional value and quality of food (Saeed *et al.*, 2012). Samples from various plant species collected in the present study, were extracted with methanol solvent in accordance with the previous report that phenolic compounds contain hydroxyl group which is most effectively soluble in high polarity solvents (Wang and Weller, 2006). In the present study, the total phenolics of selected medicinal plants show variations between them. This could be due to the presence of a diverse quantity of carotenoids, sugars, ascorbic acid and geographical variation or different extraction procedures (Burri *et al.*, 2017). The characterization of phenolic compounds is based on various phenol groups. Some of them are very reactive in neutralizing free radicals by donating a hydrogen atom or an electron, chelating metal ions in aqueous solutions (Petti and Scully, 2009). As per the earlier findings, the major phenolic compounds are gallic acid and tannic acid which were found in a phenolic fraction of *P. emblica* (Kumar *et al.*, 2006).

In plant kingdom, flavonoids are a richly diverse group of phytonutrients which contains 6,000 types and subgroups classified that depends upon their chemical structure. The flavonoid compounds including flavones, flavanones, flavan-3-ols, flavonols, isoflavones and anthocyanins were reported previously (Kozłowska and Szostak-Wegierek, 2014). Flavonoids contain various biological activities such as anti-inflammatory, anti-allergic, anticancer, antiviral, anticarcinogenic, antioxidant and other epidemiological activities (Falcone *et al.*, 2012). Ever since, flavonoids are effectively connected with food ingredients and health of human beings, the requirement of flavonoids is needed much to study from different plant sources (Kumar and Pandey, 2013).

According to earlier reports, the total flavonoid content of *C. albidum* was lower when compared to other species, against the highest flavonoid content in the present study, the variation may be due to different extraction procedures and environmental conditions (Manipal *et al.*, 2017). The present study corroborates with a previous report of that $NaNO_2$ formation a complex due to the nitration of aromatic with hydroxyl groups of flavonoid three and four positions. The acid-stable complexes were formed by aluminium chloride with C-4 or C-3 either C-5 hydroxyl group of flavonoids (Agbo *et al.*, 2015).

As per the previous reports, it was noted that the Combretaceae family is familiar for antimicrobial activity, particularly the *Combretum* genus is the most potential for the antimicrobial property (McGaw *et al.*, 2001; Fyhrquist *et al.*, 2002; Zalke *et al.*, 2013). The *C. albidum* methanolic leaf extract revealed the inhibition property against MDR *Pseudomonas aeruginosa* (Sahu *et al.*, 2014). Sreedhar *et al.* (2013) enumerated that stem bark extract of *C. albidum* has effective antibacterial activity against *K. pneumonia, E. coli, P. aeruginosa, P.mirabilis, S. typhimurium* and *B. Subtilis*. Antibacterial activity of bark and leaf extracts of *C. albidum* shows greatest inhibitory effect against seven bacterial strains, the highest zone of inhibition was found against *Pseudomonas aeruginosa* (Arundhati *et al.*, 2018). According to Chandar and Ramasamy (2016), the Gram-positive bacteria shows the highest zone of inhibition when compared to Gram-negative bacteria except for *P. mirabilis*. The plant extracts show different results may be due to different solvent extraction and the presence of bioactive components in plant materials that dissolve in the various solvent system (Mohan and Pandey, 2016; Sarita *et al.*, 2019). The antibacterial activity of selected plants in the present study shows more effective on gram positive bacteria and less inhibition on gram negative bacteria which is in accordance with the previously reported findings (Maity *et al.*, 2010; Perumal *et al.*, 2012; Al-Daihan *et al.*, 2013; Murugan *et al.*, 2013; Rubaka *et al.*, 2014, Muniyappan and Nagarajan 2014; Siddiqha *et al.*, 2017).

Free radicals are associated with many diseases such as arthritis, diabetes mellitus, cancer, aging and the antioxidant compounds found to be play a vital role in the therapy and prevention of these diseases. The antioxidants are scavenging free radicals and deal with various assays such as DPPH radical scavenging, superoxide radical scavenging, ABTS radical scavenging, hydroxyl radical scavenging, iron chelating activity, hydrogen peroxide, lipid peroxidation assay and nitric oxide scavenging assay (Soni *et al.*, 2014). Hence the present investigation carried out in the selected plant species to evaluate comparatively. Antioxidants are very much important to activate the cells healthy and play a valuable role in food products (Sharma *et al.*, 2013). Plant-based antioxidant contains different chemical diversity, the total antioxidant ability of a compound does not imitate by a single antioxidant assay. These may be happens based on the redox and synergic interactions along with various Phyto-constituents. The total antioxidant ability of plant products was improved by various methods like monitoring of terminal point and variation in different radicals or target molecules (Huang *et al.*, 2005). The action of antioxidants is based on the transfer of hydrogen atom, single electron transfer, sequential proton loss and electron transfer (Maity *et al.*, 2013). In the present study, total phenolics, reducing power for single electron transfer method and DPPH for sequential proton loss and electron transfer method was chosen to evaluate antioxidant property. Gulcin *et al.* (2004) explained that electron transfer based assays determine the reducing ability, whereas sequential proton loss and electron transfer based assays calculate the electron-donating capacity and hydrogen atom of antioxidants.

DPPH free radical accepts a proton-electron radical develop into a constant diamagnetic molecule. The reduction capability of DPPH radicals was determined by the DPPH assay which is a widely used assay to detect free radical scavenging activity of chemical components. In the earlier investigation, the *C. albidum* was extracted with ethanol and subjected to free radical scavenging test, the extract was capable to reduce and decolorize the free radicals of DPPH (Chandar and Ramasamy, 2016). The similar results were obtained in the present study which mainly due to the selective method of antioxidant testing. The presence of antioxidants in the plant extract will results in the reduction of Fe^{3+} to Fe^{2+} through contributing an electron molecule. The reduction of Fe^{3+} to Fe^{2+} complex changes information of Perl's Prussian blue was measured by at 700 nm. The maximum absorbance value indicates the highest reduction capability. The earlier studies demonstrated that antioxidant action was occurred by donating hydrogen atom in the direction to cleave the free radical chain (Nabavi *et al.*, 2008).

According to the research investigations of many scientists from various countries, phenolic compounds have been proven with the potential antioxidant ability (Kähkönen *et al.*, 1999; Saeed *et al.*, 2012; Ghasemi Pirbalouti *et al.*, 2013; Somayeh *et al.*, 2017; Aryal *et al.*, 2019). The flavonoids from *E. hirta* contain lower antioxidant capacity when compared to phenolic compounds because flavonoids are a subgroup of phenolic compounds that had a lesser antioxidant activity than phenolic compounds (Basma *et al.*, 2011). The extracts of *Z. officinale* have strong antioxidant radical activities proved by ABTS assay. However, in nature, *Z. officinale* has significant antioxidant activity hence the consumption might be prevented from oxidative stress (Morakinyo *et al.*, 2011). According to Maruthappana and Shreeb (2010), the antioxidant activity of *K. reticulata*, methanol extract shows the highest percentage of inhibition when compared to ethanol extract at higher concentrations. Whereas, the present study proves that methanol extracts show good antioxidant activity at higher concentrations. Savita (2009) reported that ethanol extract of *S. nux-vomica* acquires significant antioxidant properties without undesirable effects side effects.

Though the plant preparation is realized to use in medicinal purposes, the identification of commercial samples to find their genuineness and as certain the identity of adulterant and substituent. Therefore, the pharmacognosy study helps in identify the quality of plant preparations through its physiochemical and anatomical studies. Moreover, deficient in standardization, unprincipled mercantile preparation of adulterating and alternative natural medicines are posing a problem in popularizing time-tested traditional medicines (Sharma and Kumar, 2016). The macro- and microscopical standards of *C. albidum* stem bark was studied and reported that stem bark is typically hard and contains longitudinal cracks with 0.5 to 1 cm thickness, yellow in color, odorless and the taste was bitter. The anatomy results showed the presence of cortex, secondary phloem with phloem fibers and cork. The presence of tannin, lignin, starch grains, and oil was confirmed by histochemical studies (Sreedhar *et al.*, 2012). Zhao *et al.* (2011) enumerated that a fluorescent microscope contains ultraviolet light creates fluorescence in chemical constituents of bioproducts when it is not visible in daylight. If some of the components are not fluorescent, that kind of components are rehabilitated into fluorescent derivatives by using various reagents. Therefore, the pharmacognostic evaluation of the present study was intended to assess the qualitative and major parameters of the crude drug.

The quantitative determination of some pharmacognostic parameters is useful for setting standards for crude drugs. The quantitative determination of pharmacognostical parameters such as stomatal index value, stomatal number, palisade ratio, vein termination and vein islet is correspondingly significant evaluation of purity of drugs (Kumar *et al.*, 2011). The present results of the pharmacognostic studies were compared with previous reports of *Diospyros melanoxylon* Roxb, *Buchanani alanzan* spreng and *Manilkar azapota* (Linn.) (Bothara and Singh, 2012), *Cissus quadrangularis* L. (Nagani *et al.*, 2011), *C. albidum* G.Don (Sreedhar *et al.*, 2012), *Alternanther asessilis* L. (Anitha and Konimozhi, 2012), *Gmelina arborea* Roxb. (Acharya *et al.*, 2012) and *Eriosema chinense* Vogel (Prasad *et al.*, 2013). The microscopical parameters of the present study shows the specific structures in morphology and anatomy useful for identify of *C. albidum* drug.

The essential oil of *C. albidum* leaves was isolated by hydrodistillation method and the chemical composition was analyzed by GC/MS, in which the result shows 44 compounds and contains a complex mixture of monoterpenes and sesquiterpenes (Kumar *et al.*, 2017). Moreover, GC-MS analysis of *C. albidum* leaf oil shows 18 components (Zalke *et al.*, 2013) and ethanol leaf extract of *C. albidum* contains 23 compounds (Chandar and Ramasamy, 2016). Whereas, the present study of GC/MS result shows 14 compounds. The compound such as phytol from *C. albidum* possesses antibacterial activity (Ghaneian *et al.*, 2015), anticancer activity (Thakor *et al.*, 2016), antioxidant action (Pejin *et al.*, 2014), anti-inflammatory activity (Silva *et al.*, 2014) and antinociceptive (Santos *et al.*, 2013). The present study shows 6-methoxy flavones was one of the compound identified but, the earlier study proves that 6-methoxy flavone is a potential applicant to improve an effective immunomodulator through the suppression of NFAT-mediated T cell activation (So *et al.*, 2014). Chandar and Ramasamy (2016), demonstrated that GC-MS of *C. albidum* contains enormous presence of vitamin E, which is a powerful source of nutrition. Compounds such as stigmasterol, phytol, palmitic acid, oleic acid, and azafrin have a great responsibility for the antioxidant activities (Prachayasittikul *et al.*, 2008; Costa *et al.*, 2016; El-Agbar *et al.*, 2018; Yang *et al.*, 2018) which were identified in the present study.

Formononetin is a phytoestrogen and an O-methylated isoflavone were previously isolated from *Astragalus membranaceous* root by Yu *et al.* (2010a) which are important phytoconstituents. Isoflavones have a potential role in various diseases such as cardiovascular diseases, amelioration of postmenopausal symptoms, cognitive function and cancer (Verheus *et al.*, 2007). The nutraceuticals like isoflavone are mostly evaluated by polyphenol supplements and the isoflavones are dietary components, which is not sufficient in Western diets when compared to Asian diets because of their consumption of soya products. So, there is a need for isolation and exploration of these compounds from new plant sources (Wang *et al.*, 2013).

The interaction of model transport protein and human serum albumin with formononetin was previously studied by using FT-IR spectroscopy, fluorescence anisotropy and molecular modeling methods (Li *et al.*, 2006). Zuanazzi *et al.* (1998) observed the UV–visible spectrum of formononetin in methanol solvent contains absorption peak at 205, 215, 240 and 305 nm after that Srivastava and team (2015), found the absorption peak in solvent phase was 211, 222, 249 and 269 nm whereas, gas phase was 213, 219, 264 and 276 nm. The present study shows the peaks related to the isoflavonoid group, this is an agreement with the previous report that the FTIR spectrum of formononetin contains bands arising at 1608, 1569 and 1,513 cm^{-1} corresponds to the vibration of an aromatic compound like isoflavone group (Guo *et al.*, 2018).

In the present study, the anti-inflammatory activity of the compound CA1 was investigated on LPS-stimulated RAW 264.7 mouse macrophages, which is an accordance with previous reports, that macrophages are activated with toxins like lipopolysaccharides (LPS) initiate a cascade of inflammatory events that are mediated by a wide range of markers. LPS-stimulated macrophages produce inflammatory mediators such as free radicals, NO, iNOS, and IL-6 (Meng and Lowell *et al.*, 1997). The anti-inflammatory effects of formononetin explored the expressions of NF-κB, which response to inflammation and microglia during brain damage the dynamic immune cells obtain an immune response and astrocytes, developed neuronal damage and pro-inflammatory cytokines are produced by neural cells (Karthikeyan *et al.*, 2016). The animal bodies affected by various types of inflammatory processes due to the active role of nitric oxide was also reported. The plant extract or compound inhibited the nitrite formation by challenging through oxygen to react with nitric oxide directly and to inhibit its synthesis (Nimal Christhudas *et al.*, 2013). The analgesic and anxiolytic effects of an active compound formononetin, which is a traditional medicine of Chinese *Trifolium pratense* L. The ability to protect neurons from N-methyl-D-aspartate evoked excito toxic injury on mice suffering from complete Freund's adjuvant (CFA)-induced chronic inflammatory pain (Wang *et al.*, 2019). Formononetin resulted in the reduction of few inflammatory mediators like NF-κB and IL-1β was reported by Wang *et al.* (2012). Moreover, formononetin was capable to reduce the TNF-α and IL-6 levels and increases the superoxidase dismutase activity (Li *et al.*, 2014, Ma *et al.*, 2013). There is a way to control inflammatory conditions that is to restrain the neutrophil functions. The relationship between the traditional use of a plant compounds and an inflammatory process has been studied using several species of medicinally important plants (Suyenaga *et al.*, 2011). El-Bakoush and Olajide (2018) found that the inhibition of neuroinflammation by the NF-κB signaling pathway in LPS-activated microglia for the first time in the compound formononetin. They produce a supplementary proof on the anti-neuro inflammatory activity of the compound formononetin. The earlier reports on the inflammatory studies show that formononetin obtained from several natural sources including many plant species were reported to inhibit the nitric oxide release in LPS-stimulated RAW264.7 cells (Lai *et al.*, 2013). Moreover, bone marrow-derived dendritic cells can able to produce pro-inflammatory cytokine (Li *et al.*, 2014). Besides, formononetin has an inhibitory effect on TNF-α and NO production from microglia-enriched culture and neuronglia cultures (Chen *et al.*, 2014). Many studies reported that formononetin inhibits NF-κB in various cellular models (Wang *et al.*, 2012; Jia *et al.*, 2014; Huh *et al.*, 2014). These reports further witnessed present experimental results on the plant compounds and its anti-inflammatory activity.

The origin of cells from cervix uteri causes malignant neoplasm called as cervical cancer. The abnormal vaginal bleeding is a common symptom for cervical cancer, other than no symptoms in anticipation of cancer has developed in advanced stage (Smith *et al.*, 2013). The previous investigation reports that the two important findings pertaining to cervical cancer as the cell was inhibited by formononetin through Akt inactivation and caspase-3 activation and formononetin impaired the energy metabolism in HeLa cells (Jin *et al.*, 2013). The anticancer activity of bioactive compound CA1 isolated in the present investigation inhibited the HeLa human cervical cancer cells upto 78% at 320 µg/ml of concentration, which clearly indicates the growth inhibitory signalling mechanism on cancer cells through apoptotic activity. Numerous mechanisms have been proposed earlier, to elucidate the action of formononetin *in vitro* and *in vivo* anti-cancer activities. Ye *et al.* (2012) declared that the formononetin treated human prostate cancer cells was induced apoptosis by ERK1/2 mitogen-activated protein kinase inactivation. Auyeung *et al.* (2012), treated human colon cancer cells with formononetin and the results show significant growth-inhibitory activity and initiates the proapoptotic activity. The observation of the previous study suggested that the formononetin and multiwalled carbon-nanotube formononetin induce apoptosis which contains the highest ROS signal in HeLa cells. Moreover, the multiwalled carbon-nanotube formononetin exhibited anticancer activity that deals with ROS-mediated mitochondrial dysfunctions induced apoptosis (Guo *et al.*, 2018).

SUMMARY AND CONCLUSION

CHAPTER VI

SUMMARY AND CONCLUSION

SUMMARY

Thiruvadisoolam village of Kanchipuram district, Tamil Nadu, India was selected for the ethnobotanical survey of the present Investigation. Totally, 54 species of medicinally important plants belonging to 46 Genera and 35 families, which includes Apocynaceae (7 genera), Leguminosae (5 genera), Phyllanthaceae and Lamiaceae (3 genera each) and less than 2 genera from various other families were recorded in the survey. Most frequently, the plant leaves (24%) were widely used for various ailments by herbalists and tribal, when compared to other plant parts used.

The present study indicates that the tribal and local herbalist used various plants to cure different human diseases such as fever, skin diseases, anticancer, diabetes, vomiting, wounds, jaundice, liver diseases, leprosy, bronchitis, earache, increase sperm count in men, cardiotonic, urinary troubles, blood purification, increase the memory, anaemia, chest pain, burns, dog bites, ulcer, reduce body heat, uterus disorders, toothache and dysentery.

It was also observed that the various plant parts are used for the preparations like infusions, decoctions, fumigation, maceration, powder, cream, bath, tablets and the majority of the plants in the form of powder.

The survey conducted with 24 native herbalists, in which Men found to have the more traditional medicine knowledge when compared to women. The age group of herbalists varied with the adults from 31 to 40 age, who have more informative when compared to other age group category people. Moreover, 34% of herbalists found were illiterate.

Based on the present ethnobotanical study, the frequently used medicinally valuable and abundant plants in the area are *Carissa spinarum, Carmona retusa, Combretum albidum, Cassia auriculata, Euphorbia hirta, Gmelina asiatica, Kirganelia reticulate, Phyllanthus emblica, Strychnosnux-vomica* and *Zingiber officinale* which were selected for the present study. The above 10 plants were collected, shade dried and grinded to a fine powder. The samples from leaf and rhizome powder were extracted with methanol solvent and condensed as a sample extract for further study.

The above plant samples were examined to identify the presence of various phytoconstituents and the result shows that plants contain various phytoconstituents like phenols, alkaloids, flavonoids, glycosides, saponins, terpenoids, proteins, tannins, steroids and reducing sugars in the concentration from higher to lower level.

The total phenolic content of selected medicinal plants was measured using the Folin-Ciocalteu method. Among all the plant species, *C. albidum* contains the highest phenolic content (212.1 mg GAE/g) and *S. nux-vomica* has the lowest phenolic content (12.56 mg GAE/g). The total flavonoid content of different plant extracts was examined by aluminium chloride method and found from 8.26 to 143.06 mg QE/g. The highest flavonoid content was found in *C. albidum* (143.06 mg QE/g) and the lowest flavonoid content was found in *C. spinarum* plant (8.26 mg QE/g).

Antibacterial activity of the methanolic plant extracts was tested against two-gram positive bacteria namely *M. luteus, B. subtilis* and two-gram negative bacteria namely *S. typhi* and *P. mirabilis* against Cefalaxin as a positive control. The methanolic extract of *C. albidum* has the highest zone of bacterial growth (22mm) inhibition against *M. luteus* when compared to other plants.

The total antioxidant activity of the selected medicinal plants was observed by the Phosphomolybdenum reduction assay. The concentration of 320 μg/ml crude methanolic extract shows the highest range of absorbance value in the reduction of Phosphomolybdenum, in which *C. albidum* shows highest value as 1.36. The absorbance value of other samples ranging from 0.08 to 1.1.

The widely used DPPH method was followed to examine the capacity of compounds or complex mixtures to act as hydrogen donors or reducers of free radicals to determine the antioxidant activity. Among the methanolic plant extracts tested, *C. albidum* shows the highest radical scavenging activity (65.94 %), when compared to other plants. The study indicates that the increase in inhibition percentage of free radicals was due to an increase in extract concentration. The IC_{50} value of DPPH radical scavenging of *C. albidum* was at 147.74 µg/ml.

For the analysis of the reducing power activity of the above selected plants, it showed that a significant dose-dependent reducing activity at various concentrations. The reducing powers ability was more in *C. albidum* leaf extract than the other plant species.

The pharmacognostic study of *C. albidum* leaf was conducted to examine the quality and purity parameters of the plant. The results clearly revealed that the architectural contour of leaf and the presence of calcium oxalate crystals in the plant parts are indication of originality of the plant species.

The GC-MS analysis of methanolic leaf extract of *C. albidum* shows various compounds such as (i) Phenol 2,4-bis-(1,1-dimethylethyl), (ii) Flavone, (iii) 6-methoxy flavone, (iv) palmitic acid, (v) oleic acid, (vi) Phytol, (vii) Coumarine, 3-[2-(1-methyl-2-imidazolylthio)-1-oxoethyl], (viii) 4-(benzyloxy)-4-(2,2-dimethyl-1,3-d ioxolan-4-yl) butanal, (ix) Stigmasterol, (x) Corynan-17-ol, 18,19-didehydro-10-methoxy-, acetate (ester), (xi) Pregna-4,6-diene-3,20-dione, 17-(acetyloxy)-6-methyl, (xii) Azafrin and (xiii) 6-Bromo-1,1,4,4,7-pentamethyl-1,2,3,4-tetrahydronaphthalene, which give the information of presence of different chemical compound significant on their activity.

TLC is exploited for separation and enumeration of biocomponents in *C. albidum* methanolic extract. The solvent system hexane and ethyl acetate in the ratio of 9:1was used and the results show eight compounds which obscured as spots. Based on the TLC separation of compounds from methanol extract of *C. albidum*, column chromatography was performed on silica gel and the fractions were eluted with continuous hexane and ethyl acetate gradients. The single yellow spot was purified and isolated which might be an active biocompound involve in biological activity.

The FTIR spectrum of isolated fraction of biocompound from *C. albidum* shows various peaks which corresponds to a hydroxyl group, carbonyl group and methyl group. The

NMR spectrum of isolated fraction also was studied and found out the position and number of carbon atoms present in the molecule. The ^{13}C NMR spectrum results totally of 16 carbon atoms. Whereas, ^{1}H NMR spectrums are used to determine the position and amount of protons present in the molecule. There are totally 12 hydrogen atoms were recorded in the isolated fraction.

The isolated and purified compound (CA1) *C. albidum* was further analysed for its antioxidant property by various methods because it is a measure of cell proliferation activity. The DPPH radical scavenging activity of isolated and purified compound of *C. albidum* (CA1) significant effect in a dose-dependent manner (5- 25 µg/ml) in the reaction mixture. The results showed that the DPPH radical scavenging capacity of CA1 was moderate and that is 50% when compared with ascorbic acid which as standard. The IC_{50} value of CA1 is 13.05 µg/ml and 8.6 µg/ml for ascorbic acid.

The superoxide radical scavenging activity of CA1 and standard ascorbic acid shows nearly comparable performance as the IC_{50} of CA1 is 13.05 µg/ml and 9.46 µg/ml for ascorbic acid. The hydroxyl radical scavenging ability of CA1 and ascorbic acid shows a significant effect in a dose-dependent manner in which the IC_{50} of CA1 is 141 µg/ml and 113.73 µg/ml for ascorbic acid.

Nitric oxide radical scavenging activity of CA1 was assessed in various concentrations of sample extract and contains higher inhibition percentage with lower IC_{50} value of 30.65 µg/ml and 16.44 µg/ml for ascorbic acid. Overall the isolated compound CA1 has an effective role against oxidative stress and found to have antioxidant potential

The anti-inflammatory activity of *C. albidum* crude extract and CA1 fraction was carried out on the viability of RAW 264.7 macrophages cells by *in vitro* condition. Based on the MTT result the CA1 has exhibited moderate effect on anti-inflammatory properties. The effect of CA1 fraction on LPS-induced NO production and inducible nitric oxide synthase (iNOS) was determined. The inhibition of cells was declined up to 22% at the concentration of 320 µg/ml after 24 hrs incubation. The gene expression of iNOS and the enzyme which synthesizes NO was evaluated and found that the LPS has up-regulated the iNOS level and down-regulated in the plant treated groups.

Further, the anti-inflammatory mechanism was enumerated in detail and found the LPS stimulated the expression of pro-inflammatory cytokines TNF-α, IL- 1β and IL-10.

Hence the COX-2 was up-regulated in the LPS-induced group and gene expression of anti-inflammatory cytokine IL-10 was down-regulated.

The *in vitro* anticancer activity of CA1 and crude extract on the HeLa human cervical cancer cell line on MTT assay was carried out and the result shows the inhibition percentage of 78.32 % and 61.38% at higher concentration as 320 µg/ml respectively. The results clearly indicate that HeLa human cervical cancer cells are effectively inhibited by CA1 when compared to methanolic extract as IC_{50} value which was 108.25 µg/ml and 260.67 µg/ml, respectively.

The microscopic images of CA1 treatment on ROS generation show the increase of fluorescence intensity in a dose-dependent manner. The apoptotic induction of treated and untreated HeLa cells was labeled with Acridine Orange/ Ethidium Bromide stain and found the green fluorescence indicates the presence of live cells or untreated cells. The early-stage apoptotic cells were identified by the presence of yellow color fluorescence and the orange stained cells indicate the presence of late-stage apoptotic cells. The dead cells or necrotic cells were notified by the presence of red color cells. whereas the CA1 induces the apoptosis to 39.43% at 54 µg/ml and 80.61% at 108 µg/ml.

The flow cytometry analysis explained that the cells exposed to a significant increase in the accumulation of the DNA contents in the G0/G1phase. Both S and G2/M phase cells decreased in the treatment. It has been observed that CA1 arresting cells in the G0/G1phase of the cell cycle.

The gene expression study reveals the CA1 induced apoptosis through the promising signalling pathways. The anti-apoptotic protein Bcl-2 level was decreased, meanwhile, the pro-apoptotic proteins like Bax, caspase-3, caspase-9 and cytochrome c were increased in low dose and high dose.

CONCLUSION

The present study concludes that the medicinally important plants are essential and significant to meet the primary health care of the local people as well as in urban areas. The traditional knowledge of Thiruvadisoolam local healers and tribals found to very deep knowledge and they were highly experienced with the medicinal use of different plant species, which scientifically reflects through various pharmacological and biological experimental activities. The study has contributed to the documentation of enormous indigenous knowledge and information on medicinal plants and plant-based remedies practiced among the local people for treating and curing various common and chronic diseases. Moreover, the study proved that many plant species are useful in prenatal and postnatal healthcare and treatment of illness in infants. The results have strongly recommended that *C. albidum* plants have an effective role in antibacterial, antioxidant, anti-inflammatory and anticancer properties. The present study also evidenced for the presence of bio-compounds which belongs to particular reactive chemical groups take part in the biochemical metabolic reactions and reduce the harmful effects in cellular metabolism. This has been proved that the isolated compound 7-Hydroxy-4'-methoxy isoflavone from the plant species *C. albidum* were identified by various molecular techniques.

However, future studies like clinical trials of the purified compounds are required for exploiting the natural compounds for formulation of plant based drugs to treat various human disorders including the chronic disease like cancer.

www.ingramcontent.com/pod-product-compliance
Lightning Source LLC
Chambersburg PA
CBHW051834150726
47998CB00001B/412